NEW GENDER MAINSTREAMING SERIES ON DEVELOPMENT ISSUES

Gender Mainstreaming in HIV/AIDS

Taking a Multisectoral Approach

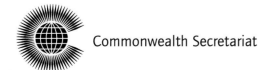

Commonwealth Secretariat

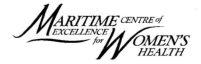

Commonwealth Secretariat
Marlborough House
Pall Mall, London SW1Y 5HX
United Kingdom

This publication was financially
supported by the Centres of
Excellence for Women's Health
Program, Women's Health Bureau,
Health Canada. The views expressed
herein do not necessarily represent
the views or the official policy of
Health Canada.

Published by the Commonwealth
Secretariat

Design: Wayzgoose
Cover design: Tony Leonard
Cover photo: Malcolm Linton
Printed in the United Kingdom
by Abacus Direct

Wherever possible, the
Commonwealth Secretariat uses
paper sourced from sustainable
forests or from sources that
minimise a destructive impact
on the environment.

Copies of this publication can
be ordered direct from:
The Publications Manager
Communication and Public
Affairs Division
Commonwealth Secretariat
Marlborough House
Pall Mall, London SW1Y 5HX
United Kingdom
Tel: +44 (0)20 7747 6342
Fax: +44 (0)20 7839 9081
E-mail:
r.jones-parry@commonwealth.int
Price: £8.99
ISBN: 0-85092-655-6

Web sites:
http://www.thecommonwealth.org/gender
http://www.thecommonwealth.org
http://www.youngcommonwealth.org

Gender Management System Series:

Gender Management System Handbook

Using Gender Sensitive Indicators: A Reference Manual for Governments and Other Stakeholders

Gender Mainstreaming in Agriculture and Rural Development: A Reference Manual for Governments and Other Stakeholders

Gender Mainstreaming in Development Planning: A Reference Manual for Governments and Other Stakeholders

Gender Mainstreaming in Education: A Reference Manual for Governments and Other Stakeholders

Gender Mainstreaming in Finance: A Reference Manual for Governments and Other Stakeholders

Gender Mainstreaming in Information and Communications: A Reference Manual for Governments and Other Stakeholders

Gender Mainstreaming in Legal and Constitutional Affairs: A Reference Manual for Governments and Other Stakeholders

Gender Mainstreaming in the Public Service: A Reference Manual for Governments and Other Stakeholders

Gender Mainstreaming in Science and Technology: A Reference Manual for Governments and Other Stakeholders

Gender Mainstreaming in Trade and Industry: A Reference Manual for Governments and Other Stakeholders

A Quick Guide to the Gender Management System

A Quick Guide to Using Gender Sensitive Indicators

A Quick Guide to Gender Mainstreaming in Development Planning

A Quick Guide to Gender Mainstreaming in Education

A Quick Guide to Gender Mainstreaming in Finance

A Quick Guide to Gender Mainstreaming in the Public Service

A Quick Guide to Gender Mainstreaming in Trade and Industry

Publication Team

Commonwealth Secretariat

Gender Mainstreaming Series Co-ordinator: Rawwida Baksh-Soodeen
Contributing Editor: Tina Johnson
Production: Rupert Jones-Parry

Guest Editorial Committee:
Lucia Kiwala, Gender and Youth Affairs Division
Janey Parris, Human Resource Development Division
Rosemarie Paul, Human Resource Development Division

Canadian Team

Leader and Senior Editor: Carol Amaratunga, Maritime Centre of Excellence
    for Women's Health
Co-editor: Sandra Bentley, Interministerial Women's Secretariat, Province of
    Prince Edward Island
Co-editor and Co-publications Co-ordinator: Jacqueline Gahagan, Dalhousie
    University

Contributing Authors:
Carol Amaratunga, Maritime Centre of Excellence for Women's Health
Sandra Bentley, Interministerial Women's Secretariat, Province of Prince
    Edward Island and the Maritime Centre of Excellence for Women's Health
Liviana Calzavara, University of Toronto
Chere Chapman, University of Toronto
Ron Colman, Genuine Progress Index for Atlantic Canada (GPI Atlantic)
Naushaba Degani, University of Toronto
Colin Dodds, Genuine Progress Index for Atlantic Canada (GPI Atlantic)
Maryanne Doherty, University of Alberta
Gordon Flowerdew, Dalhousie University
Jacqueline Gahagan, Dalhousie University
Catherine Hankins, McGill University
Lois Jackson, Dalhousie University
Stephanie Kellington, AIDS Vancouver
Donald Langille, Dalhousie University
Lynne Leonard, University of Ottawa
Carol Major, Ontario Ministry of Health
Margaret Millson, University of Toronto
Alexandra Moses, University of Toronto
Ted Myers, University of Toronto
Laura Norton, Aboriginal Health Consultant
Susan Judith Ship, Aboriginal Health Consultant
Margreth Tolson, AIDS Vancouver
Evelyn Wallace, Ontario Ministry of Health
Jeff Wilson, Genuine Progress Index for Atlantic Canada (GPI Atlantic)

Contents

Figure

Tables

Foreword

In 1996, the Commonwealth Ministers Responsible for Women's Affairs mandated the Commonwealth Secretariat to develop the concept of the Gender Management System (GMS), a holistic system-wide approach to bringing a gender perspective to bear in the mainstream of all government policies, plans and programmes. The success of the GMS depends on a broad-based partnership in society in which government consults and acts co-operatively with other key stakeholders, who include civil society and the private sector. The task of gender mainstreaming has both technical and managerial dimensions, as well as the political and socio-cultural aspects of creating equality and equity between women and men as partners in the quest for social justice. The establishment and strengthening of gender management systems and of national women's machineries was identified in the 1995 Commonwealth Plan of Action on Gender and Development.

To assist member governments in meeting their commitment to implementing the Plan of Action, the Commonwealth Secretariat has produced an 11-volume series of GMS Manuals that focus on specific sectors, from agriculture to trade and industry. The conceptual and methodological framework of the GMS is presented in the *Gender Management System Handbook*. This Manual on HIV/AIDS is the first in a new series on gender mainstreaming in critical multisectoral development issues. It is hoped that it will be used by development policy-makers, planners, field staff and others, in conjunction with other publications relating to particular national contexts. It is intended that the Manual should serve as an accessible reference manual to aid users in setting up a GMS and managing problems encountered in advancing the goal of gender equality and equity in addressing the HIV/AIDS pandemic from a multisectoral perspective.

The development of the GMS series has been a collective effort between the Commonwealth Secretariat's Gender and Youth Affairs Division and many individuals and groups. Their contributions to the thinking behind the GMS are gratefully acknowledged. In particular, I would like to thank the following:

all those member governments who supported the development of the GMS and encouraged us to move the project forward; participants at the first GMS meeting in Britain in February 1996 and at the GMS Workshop in Malta in April 1998, who provided valuable input and feedback; and the Steering Committee on the Plan of Action (SCOPA). The concept for this specific co-publication on Gender Mainstreaming in HIV/AIDS arose during a Commonwealth Secretariat GMS and Health Sector Workshop in Halifax, Canada in November 1999. In accordance with the spirit and principles of a broad-based partnership, the Canadian partners and Commonwealth Secretariat jointly identified the need for a dynamic publication to enhance the capacity of governments to adopt gender-based principles in the campaign against the HIV/AIDS pandemic.

I am most grateful to Dr Carol Amaratunga and the Canadian editorial team, Dr Jacqueline Gahagan and Sandra Bentley, for their contributions to the text of this manual; to the Canadian authors; to Tina Johnson, Contributing Editor; to members of the Guest Editorial Committee; and to the staff of the Gender Affairs Department, Gender and Youth Affairs Division, particularly Dr Rawwida Baksh-Soodeen, GMS Series Co-ordinator, who conceptualised and guided the series through to publication. I also wish to acknowledge the significant contribution of The Women's Health Bureau, Health Canada in enabling this co-publication and in contributing a number of key resources, supporting case studies and partnership funding.

We share a common commitment to reducing the incidence and suffering caused by HIV/AIDS around the world and hope that this Manual will be of genuine use to you in your efforts to mainstream gender in this area.

Nancy Spence
Director, Gender and Youth Affairs Division
Commonwealth Secretariat

Preface

In November 1999, during a Commonwealth GMS and Health Sector Workshop hosted by Health Canada in Halifax, Nova Scotia, Canada, the idea for a co-publication on Gender Mainstreaming in HIV/AIDS first emerged. We are extremely grateful for the funding support and commitment of the Women's Health Bureau, Health Canada, throughout the co-publication's development.

In July 2000, the project was further expanded to include the concept of a 'transformative' International Institute on Gender and HIV/AIDS. When it comes on stream in 2003, the training institute – to be co-hosted by the Maritime (Atlantic) Centre of Excellence for Women's Health (Dalhousie University and the IWK Health Centre) and the Commonwealth Secretariat – will provide comprehensive gender training in HIV/AIDS for Commonwealth country middle-level managers and 'change agents'. The Institute will enable participants from government, voluntary and clinical sectors to design and deliver gender-sensitive approaches to national HIV/AIDS policy in the campaign against the pandemic. This co-publication is intended to serve as the 'jewel in the crown' – the first in a series of core curriculum reference materials for the Institute.

To assess the feasibility of the Institute, an International Design Workshop on Gender and HIV/AIDS was convened in Halifax, Canada by the project partners, 16–18 January 2002. We are very grateful to the Women's Health Bureau and International Affairs Directorate, Health Canada; the International Development Research Agency (IDRC) and the Canadian Institutes of Health Research (CIHR) for their generous contributions to this initiative. Thirty-one participants from 10 countries participated in the workshop and endorsed the concept of an international training institute. These participants also pledged their personal commitment to advance the International Institute on Gender and HIV/AIDS from concept to reality.

We are also most grateful to Nancy Spence, Director of the Gender and Youth Affairs Division of the Commonwealth

Secretariat, and to Dr Rawwida Baksh-Soodeen, GMS Series Co-ordinator, for their personal commitment, leadership and support for this co-publication and the training initiative. We wish to extend our sincere thanks to the Commonwealth Secretariat, IDRC, the CIHR and to Health Canada's International Affairs Directorate and Women's Health Bureau for the opportunity to participate in the global HIV/AIDS campaign through this co-publication and the International Design Workshop on Gender and HIV/AIDS. We are also grateful to the Canadian authors, peer review group and editorial team for their time, dedication and commitment in preparing this co-publication. Special thanks to Tina Johnson, Contributing Editor, for her contributions, synthesis and patient editing of the final version.

Carol Amaratunga
Executive Director
Jacqueline Gahagan
Deputy Director
Sandra Bentley
Co-Chair, Steering Committee
Maritime Centre of Excellence for Women's Health
(Dalhousie University and IWK Health Centre)

Executive Summary

Introduction

Current estimates show that 40 million people were living with HIV in December 2001 and 3 million died from HIV/AIDS-related causes during that year. 24.8 million people died from HIV/AIDS between the beginning of the pandemic and the end of December 2001. Sub-Saharan Africa is by far the worst affected region in the world, but AIDS is also the leading cause of death in the Caribbean for those aged 15–45 and the number of cases is doubling every two or three years. Asia, where more people live than any other region, is seeing alarming increases in the number of infections.

While AIDS was originally diagnosed in homosexual men, there has been a progressive shift towards heterosexual transmission as the epidemic has spread, and increasing infection rates in women. Almost as many women as men are now dying of HIV/AIDS, but the age patterns of infection vary significantly between the two sexes. Looking beyond the statistics, important differences can be identified in the underlying causes and consequences of HIV/AIDS infections in men and women, which stem from biology, sexual behaviour, social attitudes and pressures, economic power and vulnerability. These result in different rates of risk, infection patterns, access to health knowledge and protection, intervention and care management of illness.

Efforts to contain the spread of HIV/AIDS challenge governments and communities to develop policies and programmes that meet the needs of the entire population, including those who are less able to respond to the threat or consequences of infection because of social, economic or gender disadvantage. Education and treatment approaches that do not take into account gender, cultural or social disparities do not use resources efficiently or effectively and are failing to improve long-term population health outcomes. With health systems stretched far beyond their limits by the pandemic, it is vital that the meagre resources available are used in a cost-effective and equitable way. Action must be taken to ensure that women and girls have adequate access to sexual and reproductive health services and that there is equality in the provision of drugs for treating HIV/AIDS and opportunistic infections and of care to those infected.

At the same time, it has been recognised that HIV/AIDS is not solely a health problem. To successfully address the pandemic, a gender perspective has to be mainstreamed into a broad-based and multisectoral response. The notion of 'gender' as distinct from 'sex' refers to the socially constructed roles, behaviours and expectations associated with men and women. Gender roles vary depending on the particular socio-economic, political and cultural context and help to determine women's access to rights, resources and opportunities. Gender analysis – a tool that uses sex and gender as a way of conceptualising information – helps to reveal and clarify women's and men's different social relationships and realities, life expectations and economic circumstances.

Gender analysis involves the collection and use of sex-disaggregated data that reveals the roles and responsibilities of women and men. It is crucial to understanding HIV/AIDS transmission and initiating appropriate programmes of action, and forms the basis for the changes required to enable women and men to protect themselves and each other. Gender analysis provides a framework for analysing and developing policies, programmes and legislation, and is thus an important tool for gender mainstreaming.

Gender mainstreaming is the most efficient and equitable way of using existing resources for combating HIV/AIDS by focusing on the real needs of the whole population. It is also required to implement a number of international and Commonwealth mandates. The ultimate goal of gender mainstreaming is to achieve gender equality. It requires that both men's and women's concerns are considered in the design, implementation, monitoring and evaluation of policies and programmes in all political, economic and societal spheres so that women and men benefit equally. Gender mainstreaming does not, however, automatically remove the need for women-specific programmes or for projects targeting women, which will often remain necessary to redress particular instances of past discrimination or long-term, systemic discrimination.

Because gender mainstreaming cuts across government sectors and involves other social partners, it requires strong leadership and organisation. The Commonwealth approach to gender mainstreaming is through the Gender Management System (GMS). The GMS is an integrated network of structures, mechanisms and processes put in place in an existing organisational framework in order to guide, plan, monitor and evaluate the process of mainstreaming gender into all areas of an organisation's work. It is intended to advance gender equality and equity through promoting political will; forging a partnership of stakeholders including government, private sector and civil society; building capacity; and sharing good practice.

The goal of a GMS for HIV/AIDS is to ensure the integration of gender into all government policies, programmes and activities that impact on the epidemic. Within the GMS, the design, implementation, monitoring and evaluation of such policies and programmes should not only ensure equality and justice for all regardless of sex and gender, but should also take into account the contributions that can be made by all stakeholders working in the area.

A Gender Analysis of HIV/AIDS

In most societies, gender relations are characterised by an unequal balance of power between men and women, with women having fewer legal rights and less access to education, health services, training, income-generating activities and property. This situation affects both their access to information about HIV/AIDS and the steps that they can take to prevent its transmission.

Both men and women are subject to ideas about what is normal behaviour for one or the other sex, what are 'typical' feminine and masculine characteristics, and about how women and men should act in particular situations. For example, men are generally expected to be more knowledgeable than women about sex, which can make them reluctant to seek information. Women may also have limited access to information about HIV/AIDS, sexuality and reproductive health because of social pressures and cultural norms that stress their innocence. Cultural beliefs and expectations tend to make men responsible for deciding when, where and how sex will take place, while women generally lack control over sex and reproduction. This heightens not only women's but also men's vulnerability to HIV and other sexually transmitted infections (STIs).

Many societies share the idea that women seduce men into having sex and that men cannot resist because their sexual needs are so strong. All over the world, men are expected to have more sex partners than women, including more extra-marital partners, a tendency reinforced by male migration and mobility. Such beliefs and practices are an obstacle to HIV/AIDS prevention because they absolve men from taking responsibility for their sexual behaviour. They also mean that women are more likely to be infected by their steady male partner.

The feminisation of poverty has meant that women and girls are increasingly having to exchange sex for money, food, shelter or other needs, and that much of this sex is unsafe. They are also vulnerable to being trafficked into sexual slavery. Women may also be blamed as the vectors of the disease since they are often the ones who are tested (when they are pregnant). This can lead to discrimination and stigma. The cultural expectation that women will be the prime or only care-givers to their infected family members creates disproportionate social and economic burdens on them. The costs of medicines and treatment are very high, reducing families' abilities to pay for education and other services. Sickness and death cause labour shortages that increase food insecurity.

There are also harmful traditional and customary practices that make women and girls more vulnerable to HIV infection. These include early marriage, wife inheritance, wife cleansing, dry sex and female genital mutilation (FGM). Gender-based violence also increases the risk of HIV/AIDS. The most pervasive form is that committed against a woman by her intimate partner, often connected to marital rape, coerced sex or other forms of abuse that lead to HIV transmission. Gender-based violence is particularly prevalent in armed conflicts. The main perpetrators are military personnel, who tend to have much higher rates of STIs – which can increase the risk of HIV infection – than the civilian population.

Both women and men need to be empowered to protect themselves against HIV/AIDS. Women need information and education, skills, access to services and technologies, access to economic resources, social capital and the opportunity to have a voice in decision-making at all levels. Men need to become partners in prevention and education, and to be encouraged to adopt healthier sexual behaviour. This means that in addition to health information, education, counselling and services, they should be provided with information about the gender dimensions of HIV/AIDS and the implications of their behaviour for women, families and communities.

In many of the heavily affected countries, young people are the most rapidly growing group of new HIV/AIDS infections, with girls far outnumbering boys. Some of the reasons for this are related to poverty, lack of information, lack of economic and social empowerment and lack of availability of protective methods. Many countries offer no sexual and reproductive health services to adolescents. Even where such services do exist, they may be hard to access for a number of reasons.

Young women and men are establishing their sexual and gender identities, and face various pressures in this area from their peers and from society as a whole. Young women often have less decision-making power regarding sexuality than adult women, especially because they tend to have older male partners. While young men may be expected to be aggressive, in control of sexual relationships and sexually knowledgeable, young women may be expected to be passive as well as innocent about sexual matters. Young men are often encouraged to start having sex from an early age and to have a number of different partners to prove their manhood. Young women are particularly vulnerable because their immature genital tracts may tear during sexual activity, creating a greater risk of HIV transmission. This is especially likely during forced sex.

Young people are the key to controlling the HIV/AIDS epidemic since adolescence is the critical time for intervention to ensure that high-risk sexual behaviour patterns do not become entrenched. Behaviour begun in adolescence affects the current and future health of the individual and the population as a whole. An important first step would be to acknowledge that many young men and women are sexually active and thus need to receive sex education. Far from sex education promoting promiscuity, numerous studies have found that it is ignorance that increases vulnerability to infection. When young people have information about sex, they tend to delay sexual intercourse or use condoms. Young people should also play a central role in AIDS prevention and care programmes, and strategies need to be developed that utilise their energies and expertise.

A Multisectoral Response to HIV/AIDS

Since HIV/AIDS is not just a health issue but is affected by and impacts on every aspect of life, it is vital that it is met by a multisectoral response. This response must be dynamic and react to the epidemic as it evolves. It calls for strong and creative leadership, including political will at the highest level. Governments must take the lead in fostering a supportive environment and providing a framework for action that works both horizontally (with government, business and civil society organisations) and vertically (at international, national and community levels).

Every level of society should be involved, and partnerships need to be developed between ministries responsible for different sectors, and between them and the private sector, civil society organisations, communities and people living with HIV/AIDS. Different partners bring different strengths and experiences of partnership development, and best practice in multisectoral responses need to be shared.

Since the pattern of HIV transmission and the stage of the epidemic are different in each country, depending on the underlying social, economic, political and cultural context, a consensus needs to be reached of what needs to be done in that particular country. In preparing culturally-appropriate national HIV/AIDS policy guidelines, case studies, tools and resources, government analysts and decision-makers need to factor in gender indicators. The Gender Management System is flexible enough to be adapted to the issue of HIV/AIDS and to the distinctive national context.

Mainstreaming gender calls for skills in gender analysis and planning; the capacity to collect and interpret sex-disaggregated data; a commitment by government to action to achieve gender equality; and the availability of human, technical and financial resources. Both short- and long-term gender-sensitive strategies need to be developed from the community to the national level. Short-term strategies might focus on people's immediate needs, such as information, support to home-based care and access to treatment for STIs. More long-term strategies need to address the underlying social and cultural structures that sustain gender inequality.

In all areas, programmes have to deal with issues of economic power imbalances, migrations, economic and social marginalisation, development of community responses, participation and capacity building for sustainability. It should be recognised that education has a key role to play as a means of imparting the knowledge and skills essential for individual, communal and national survival. Any successful response will integrate prevention and care. It is not enough to focus on individual behaviour change because poor health, gender, poverty and other factors also play an important role in vulnerability and susceptibility to HIV. The poorest and most vulnerable groups, including women and young people, need to be seen as resources and not just victims.

Each sector must plan and make available resources for an integrated response, including an analysis of the factors within the sector that contribute to the spread of HIV/AIDS, the impact of the disease on its workforce and products, and the consequences for both the sector and the community. Practical short-term and long-term interventions need to be developed to protect the sector's workers, to cope with the skills shortages that will arise and to mitigate the adverse effects on society.

In **agriculture**, for example, it is likely that the AIDS epidemic will cause a major labour shortage in many countries. If a family member is sick with AIDS, it will usually be a woman who cares for them, meaning she may be unable to carry out her usual agricultural tasks. This in turn may result in chronic food insecurity as well as high levels of malnutrition and micro-nutrient deficiencies. Girls may also be kept out of school to care for the sick or help with household tasks.

In addition, the deaths of farmers, extension workers and teachers from AIDS can undermine the transmission of knowledge and know-how as well as the local capacity to absorb technology transfers. Widows may be left without access to productive resources such as land, credit and technology and their livelihoods may be threatened. HIV/AIDS also leads to a reduction in investment in irrigation, soil enhancement and other capital improvements.

HIV/AIDS not only affects **education** through the loss of

personnel, reduction of available government resources and decline in demand. It also exacerbates the gender-based disparities that already exist in the education sector, which in most cases disadvantage girls in their access to quality education and women in their employment opportunities as educators and administrators.

Schools need to play a positive role in helping learners and teachers to cope with the issue of HIV/AIDS. They can influence social attitudes and cultural norms acquired by young people. Schools can also play an important role as focal points for the community. Teachers, parent-teacher associations and governing bodies often command a degree of respect and authority that can be used to advantage in mobilising community action. Schools also need to produce an adequate supply of educated people with the skills and training needed to support themselves, their families and communities against a background where there are increasing human resource shortages due to the devastating impact of HIV/AIDS.

The epidemic has had a profound impact on **health** services in most of the affected countries, with more people requiring hospital care at the same time that there are reduced numbers of health staff. Treatments for controlling HIV, such as triple, double or combination antiretroviral therapy are often prohibitively expensive. Yet a single dose of an antiretroviral given to an infected woman in labour, and another dose given to her baby within three days of birth, could prevent some 300,000 to 400,000 babies per year being born infected with HIV.

If costly drugs are unobtainable, people living with HIV/AIDS must at least have access to basic pain relief and treatment for 'simpler' opportunistic infections such as pneumonia and tuberculosis. Care and support for people living with HIV/AIDS can help to protect the health of the rest of the population by making prevention more effective.

HIV/AIDS brings about reduced **labour** quality and supply, more frequent and longer periods of absenteeism, and losses in skills and experience. This results in a younger, less experienced workforce and causes production losses. Women who become HIV positive are more likely than men to lose employment in the formal sector and to face discrimination and even expulsion from their homes. When they are forced to become the main breadwinner due to their partner becoming infected, women who lack education and skills may be forced into hazardous occupations, including sex work, that further increase their vulnerability.

HIV/AIDS is exacerbating the difficulties that women face in the area of **law and justice**. In many countries, women experience substantial discrimination in this area and may lack the right to hold, inherit or dispose of property, to participate in democratic processes, or to make decisions about marriage or about the education of their children. When they or their partner become HIV positive, it may be difficult for them to exercise their rights to their property, employment, marital status and security. More women are now being widowed at a younger age and may be disinherited by the husband's relatives and unable to support themselves. They may also expect to die early themselves, yet be unable to provide for their children

Laws are needed that actively promote a supportive environment. These include those that protect the right to privacy; provide redress in the event of discrimination in employment, housing, access to health care, etc.; ban discrimination against people with HIV or their family or friends; protect the confidentiality of a person's HIV status; and require consent for HIV testing.

Case Studies, Tools and Resources

The case studies illustrate how programmes that promote HIV prevention by addressing gender and the social and economic factors that increase people's risk of infection are more likely to succeed in changing behaviour. It is particularly important to listen to women's voices and address their lived realities in developing HIV/AIDS prevention campaigns. Research on HIV/AIDS that is carried out in co-operation with local communities has considerable potential to influence national policy and promote action on the social factors that affect women's and men's health and wellbeing. This increases the likelihood of being able to target strategic interventions to high-risk populations.

These populations include sex workers, and one of the case studies looks at female prostitutes and HIV prevention programmes in Canada. Other case studies from Canada include one on HIV counselling and testing among pregnant women, which offers an example of best practices in this area, and one on gender differences in sexual health promotion among adolescents.

Two case studies come from Africa. The first looks at marketing the female condom in Zimbabwe and suggests that female condoms are providing new and additional STI/HIV protection to some study participants, though more research is needed. The second describes an innovative mechanism for the transfer of local knowledge for HIV programming in Southern Africa called the 'School Without Walls'.

Involving men in preventing gender violence and HIV transmission is the focus of an international case study of a programme called 'Stepping Stones'. This uses peer groups to help people translate information about prevention into behavioural change. The need to mobilise the community for effective control and prevention is also emphasised by a case study on sexual and reproductive health integration in Bangladesh.

A final chapter on tools and resources includes a checklist that aims to provide HIV/AIDS educators and policy-makers with a tool to assess the gender sensitivity of their programmes and policies, and an extensive list of online resources.

1. Introduction

Scope and Objectives of this Manual

This reference Manual provides an overview of some of the major gender issues in the HIV/AIDS pandemic and offers suggestions for a multisectoral response. It is intended to enhance the capacity of Commonwealth countries in both the South and the North to develop gender-sensitive national HIV/AIDS strategies, programmes and policies. It encourages the building and fostering of community, government, clinical and academic partnerships which respect the perspectives and needs of people living with HIV/AIDS (PLHA). It also aims to assist countries in establishing ongoing and upgraded national monitoring and evaluation mechanisms to review past and present programming initiatives and policy directions related to HIV/AIDS prevention, care, treatment and support. It outlines some of the main issues in a variety of sectors and makes recommendations for future programme and policy priorities that are inclusive of HIV/AIDS stakeholder groups.

A primary objective of the Manual is to demonstrate the application of gender-based knowledge in the campaign against the HIV/AIDS pandemic. It uses case studies infused with the social, economic, cultural and gender dimensions of health that are relevant to individuals, families and communities. The factors affecting health outcomes involve many spheres, including genetic and biological, and social and economic conditions, the environment, individual choices and behaviours, as well as gender. Selected to display the influences and significance of relations between the sexes, the studies provide insights into the dynamic interplay between biology, gender and culture; the challenges and benefits of accommodation for numerous determinants of health; and the dynamics of promoting changes in health outcomes. A list of HIV/AIDS websites and a gender-sensitivity checklist provide ways of accessing more information and an example of a policy tool. Appendices include UN guidelines on HIV-related human rights and some of the global and Commonwealth mandates

The factors affecting health outcomes involve many spheres, including genetic and biological, and social and economic conditions, the environment, individual choices and behaviours, as well as gender.

At the end of 2001, UNAIDS and WHO estimated that the number of people living with HIV had grown to 40 million and there were 3 million deaths due to HIV/AIDS-related causes during that year.

that call on governments to take action to develop gender-inclusive education, policies and programmes for HIV/AIDS prevention and intervention. There is an extensive bibliography.

The Manual is the first in a new series on gender mainstreaming in critical development issues. This new series is an offshoot of the internationally recognised 11-volume series of Gender Management System manuals that focused on specific sectors. The GMS is explained most fully in the *Gender Management System Handbook*. An important objective of all these publications is to assist governments in advancing gender equality in their countries. However, they are also intended to be of use to other stakeholders that are involved in determining and formulating policy, applying it and ensuring its enforcement. These include international and regional agencies, the academic community, NGOs, other non-state organisations, and individual gender experts and trainers. The Manual specifically promotes the participation and inclusion of NGOs and community consultation in the development of HIV/AIDS policies, plans and programme delivery.

The Manual is also intended to serve as core curriculum reference material for the International Institute on Gender and HIV/AIDS – a partnership programme of the Maritime Centre of Excellence for Women's Health (Dalhousie University and the IWK Health Centre) and the Commonwealth Secretariat.

HIV/AIDS: An Overview

The incidence of and risk factors for HIV/AIDS worldwide

The number of HIV/AIDS cases continues to grow throughout the world despite efforts to distribute information on avoidance and/or management of risk behaviours and situations. At the end of 2001, UNAIDS and the World Health Organisation (WHO) estimated that the number of people living with HIV had grown to 40 million and there were 3 million deaths due to HIV/AIDS-related causes during that year (see Table 1). The cumulative number of deaths attributed to HIV/AIDS in the period from the onset of the pandemic to December 2001 stood at 24.8 million. AIDS is now the fourth

Table 1: Global HIV/AIDS Statistics, December 2001

		2001	1996
People newly infected with HIV	Total	5,000,000	3,100,000
	Adults	4,300,000	2,700,000
	Women	1,800,000	(no. unavailable)
	Children	800,000	400,000
People living with HIV/AIDS	Total	40,000,000	22,600,000
	Adults	37,200,000	21,800,000
	Women	17,600,000	9,200,000
	Children	2,700,000	830,000
Total AIDS deaths since the beginning of the epidemic	Total	24,800,000	6,400,000
	Adults	19,900,000	5,000,000
	Women	10,100,000	2,100,000
	Children	4,900,000	1,400,000

Source: UNAIDS/WHO, 2001.

biggest killer in the world, after heart disease, stroke and respiratory disease, and kills more people than any other infectious disease.

Sub-Saharan Africa remains by far the worst affected – and most poorly resourced – region in the world. More than 28 million Africans are HIV positive and a further 17 million have already died of AIDS. The death toll claimed by the epidemic in 2000 was ten times that caused by the region's wars and civil conflicts (UNAIDS, 2001b). If current trends do not change, there will be more than 40 million AIDS orphans in Africa by 2010 (Human Rights Watch, 2001a). In the Caribbean, according to the Director of the Caribbean Epidemiology Centre, AIDS is the leading cause of death for people aged 15–45 and the number of cases is doubling every two or three years (De Young, 2001). Asia, where more people live than any other region, is seeing alarming increases in the number of infections (see Table 2).

While AIDS was originally diagnosed in homosexual men in the USA, and there is still a widespread belief in industrialised countries that it is a 'gay disease', the first case in a woman was actually identified a mere two months after that in a man. By 1991, "AIDS was the leading killer of young women in most large US cities" (Farmer, 1999). Factors in the spread of the disease include risky behaviour such as sharing drug-

Table 2: Regional HIV/AIDS Statistics, December 2001

Region	Adults and children living with HIV/AIDS	Adults and children newly infected with HIV/AIDS	Adult prevalence rate (%)	Percentage of HIV-positive people who are female (%)
Sub-Saharan Africa	28,100,000	3,400,000	8.4	55
North Africa & Middle East	440,000	80,000	0.2	40
South Asia & South-East Asia	6,100,000	800,000	0.6	35
East Asia & Pacific	1,000,000	270,000	0.1	20
Latin America	1,400,000	130,000	0.5	30
Caribbean	420,000	60,000	2.2	50
Eastern Europe & Central Asia	1,000,000	250,000	0.5	20
Western Europe	560,000	30,000	0.3	25
North America	940,000	45,000	0.6	20
Australia & New Zealand	15,000	500	0.1	10
TOTAL	40,000,000	5,000,000	1.2	48

Source: UNAIDS/WHO, 2001.

injection equipment, transfusion of blood that is HIV infected, an injection with an unsterilised needle, and exposure to HIV in the womb or during birth or breastfeeding. However, the source of infection for the majority of people is sexual inter-course.

Worldwide, the populations now being most affected by HIV/AIDS are those socially and/or economically margin-alised by income, employment, ethnicity, culture and gender. HIV/AIDS spreads most rapidly when civil and political rights are violated. It flourishes "where women are unable to negoti-ate the terms of their sexual relations, where gay men and sex workers are marginalised and excluded from services, and where sexual violence is prevalent" (Human Rights Watch, 2001b). The Executive Director of UNFPA has stressed the fact that, "HIV, in poor and rich countries alike, is linked to discrimination, poverty, and insecurity as well as a culture of silence about the disease and refusal to take preventive action" (Obaid, 2001).

Inequality and marginalisation put people at greater risk of infection, isolation and bearing an excessive share of the responsibility for caring for self and others, as well as of pre-mature death. In industrialised countries, where antiretroviral therapy is helping HIV-positive people to live productive lives,

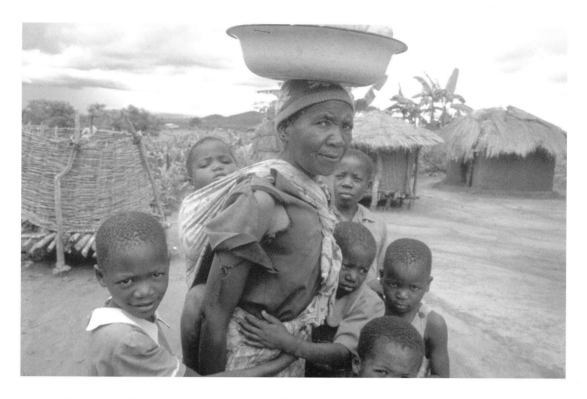

the epidemic is shifting towards poorer people, especially ethnic minorities. In Canada, for example, those at high risk of becoming HIV positive may represent 'hard to reach' or 'forgotten' populations who are excluded from the mainstream. Since 1984, the number of AIDS cases among aboriginal Canadians has risen steadily – most alarmingly among women and those under 30 (Dodds et al., 2001) (see Box 1).

The major challenge for governments and communities is to develop policies and programmes that meet the needs of the entire population. Education and treatment approaches which neglect gender, cultural or social disparities have little effect at the individual level and may be unsustainable at the policy level because they are failing to improve long-term health outcomes. Methods of intervention that do not recognise and address these inequalities fail to use resources efficiently or effectively to ameliorate underlying conditions. Such inequalities contribute to the development of epidemics and are likely to affect their enduring presence.

In Malawi, 65-year-old Maritas Shaba stands with six of the nine grandchildren whose guardian she has become since the death of both their parents from AIDS.
UNICEF/HQ93-2043/
Cindy Andrew

Box 1: HIV/AIDS and Aboriginal Women in Canada

Aboriginal women are over-represented in HIV/AIDS statistics in Canada. Research shows that those at greatest risk of HIV are most likely to be the products of families and communities devastated by the long-term effects of cultural disruption (including residential schooling) and multigenerational abuse. These factors, combined with widespread poverty, racism, sexism and the loss of traditional ways of life, have given rise to a range of pressing social problems that include alcoholism, substance abuse, high suicide rates, violence against women and family violence.

First Nations women living with HIV/AIDS experience gender discrimination as women in addition to the stigma that HIV-positive men face. Women's social role as primary caregivers and nurturers in the family constitutes a fundamental difference in their experience of HIV/AIDS compared to that of men. Aboriginal women living with HIV/AIDS are more likely to be single parents, living below the poverty line and responsible for the health and wellbeing of their children, in addition to their own, with fewer resources. Aboriginal women assume the burden of caregiving for Aboriginal people with HIV/AIDS with few supports. High rates of sexually transmitted infections (STIs), alcoholism and substance abuse, together with low rates of condom use and high rates of teenage pregnancy, continue to increase vulnerability to HIV, particularly among Aboriginal young people, who are also over-represented in high-risk groups, such as runaways, sex trade workers and intravenous drug users.

Source: Ship and Norton, 2001

Why gender and HIV/AIDS?

Mariah, a 35-year-old with three young children, found out that she was HIV positive because her husband became ill and they went for a test together. When he subsequently died and his relatives insisted she be inherited by one of his brothers, she informed them of her HIV-positive status. She was then accused of killing their son and forced out of their residence without her children.

Summarised from Nath, 2001a

An examination of the realities of women's and men's lives reveals variations in personal, physical, social and economic powers and capacities. These differences are expressed at many levels of human activities and result in differential rates of risk, infection patterns, access to health knowledge and protection, intervention and management of illness.

Across the world, there has been a changing pattern in rates of male/female HIV/AIDS infections. As the epidemic has spread there has been a progressive shift towards heterosexual transmission and increasing infection rates in women. Today, more women than men are dying of HIV/AIDS, and the age patterns of infection are significantly different for the two sexes. In sub-Saharan Africa women constitute 55 per cent of all HIV infected adults, while teenage girls are infected at a rate five to six times greater than their male counterparts (Commission on the Status of Women, 2001). In the Caribbean, women made up half of those newly infected in 2001.

In Tanzania, the third of three wives in an area where polygamy is common is left to care for all the offspring after her husband and his two other wives died of AIDS.
UNAIDS/Louise Gubb

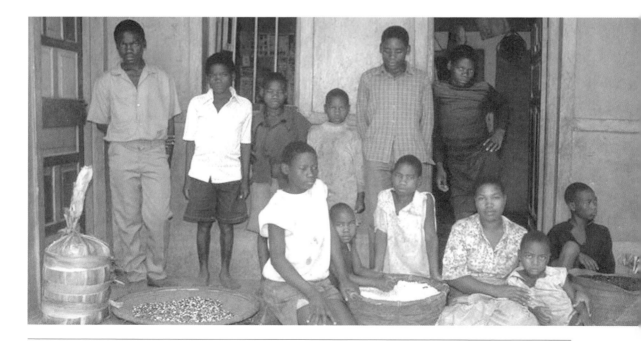

Box 2: Women's Vulnerability to HIV/AIDS

Although HIV/AIDS affects both men and women, women are more vulnerable for biological, epidemiological and social reasons:

- Women are more susceptible to HIV infection because of the vulnerability of the reproductive tract tissues to the virus, especially in young women.

- Men and women have a greater risk of acquiring HIV in the presence of sexually transmitted infections (STIs). STIs in women are less noticed and often go undiagnosed. The stigma of STIs in women can also discourage them from getting treatment.

- Cultural, social and economic pressures make women more likely to contract HIV infection than men. Women are often less able to negotiate safer sex due to factors such as their lower status, economic dependence and fear of violence.

- There is a big difference in attitudes towards men's and women's sexuality before or outside marriage. Promiscuity in men is often condoned and sometimes encouraged, while it is usually frowned upon in women.

- Young women and girls are increasingly being targeted for sex by older men seeking safe partners and also by those who erroneously believe that a man infected with HIV/AIDS can get rid of the disease by having sex with a virgin.

- Women and girls tend to bear the main burden of caring for sick family members, and often have less care and support when they themselves are infected.

- Women known to have HIV/AIDS are more likely to be rejected, expelled from the family home and denied treatment, care and basic human rights.

- There is a strong gender difference in the age-related prevalence of HIV/AIDS, with the average age of infected women in Africa typically being several years lower than that of men.

Source: Matlin and Spence, 2000

Beyond the statistics of sex-based differences in infection rates, there are profound differences in the underlying causes and consequences of HIV/AIDS infections in men and women, reflecting differences in biology, sexual behaviour, social attitudes and pressures, economic power and vulnerability (see Box 2). In general, male–female transmission of HIV is more efficient than female–male transmission, both because infected semen contains a higher concentration of the virus than female sexual secretions and because the exposed surface area of women's reproductive tract tissue is larger than the vulnerable surface area in men (Kumar, Larkin and Mitchell, 2001). Gender analysis of past attempts to address HIV/AIDS reveals significant sex and gender differences in the patterns of infection and access to information, prevention, treatment and care-giving supports. It is common in all cultures that responsibilities for management of sexual behaviour and sexual health are affected by gender. There is evidence that health promotion efforts everywhere are limited by conditions related to poverty, with high-risk behaviours and literacy levels severely reducing the delivery of health information.

It is now widely recognised that gender-based inequalities in the treatment of women and men permeate health systems in all parts of the world and this situation is mirrored in the specific area of HIV/AIDS. Examples of gender biases can be found in women's access to services for diagnosis, counselling and treatment; in the training of health professionals and their responses to patients; and in the nature and focus of research into new drugs and treatments, including the greatly disproportionate use of men as research subjects to establish the pharmacological effects and efficacy of drugs.

Redressing these biases is not simple. Countries have been struggling for years with health sector reforms in response to a variety of external and internal forces, including structural adjustment, globalisation, economic contraction and shrinkage of state support for the social sector. As of December 2000, 95 per cent of all AIDS cases have occurred in developing countries (UNAIDS, 2001a), and health systems that were previously fragile are now being stretched far beyond their limits by the pandemic. It is therefore vital to ensure that the meagre resources available are used in a cost-effective and equitable way. Culturally appropriate gender-based strategies

. . . there are profound differences in the underlying causes and consequences of HIV/AIDS infections in men and women, reflecting differences in biology, sexual behaviour, social attitudes and pressures, economic power and vulnerability.

HIV/AIDS is not solely a health problem but requires a more broadly based response going beyond biomedical models.

have been clearly shown by Canadian case study economic analyses to be highly cost effective, producing enormous savings in direct health care costs and retained productive capacity (Dodds et al., 2001). Action must be taken to ensure that women and girls have adequate access to sexual and reproductive health services and that there is equality in the provision of drugs for treating HIV/AIDS and opportunistic infections and care of those infected.

At the same time, it has been recognised that HIV/AIDS is not solely a health problem but requires a more broadly based response going beyond biomedical models. At the international level, the Joint United Nations Programme on HIV/AIDS (UNAIDS) was established in 1996. More recently, at the regional level, the UNAIDS co-sponsors and other partners have initiated an International Partnership on HIV/AIDS in Africa and the World Bank has launched its strategy on Intensifying Action Against HIV/AIDS in Africa. In the Caribbean, a regional government coalition has been launched to fight the epidemic (see Box 3). At the national level, many governments have adopted a multisectoral approach to addressing the pandemic, with the involvement of many government departments, NGOs and the private sector.

To successfully address the HIV/AIDS pandemic, a gender perspective has to be mainstreamed into these broad-based and multisectoral responses. Taking gender into account when designing policy promotes the development of options to accommodate sex and gender differences. It also brings to light cultural and economic differences, how gender roles affect the responsibilities of women and men, as well as current deficits in gender-related data and information.

A Gender Framework

What is the difference between sex and gender?

"'Gender' refers to socially constructed roles of women and men ascribed to them on the basis of their sex, whereas the term 'sex' refers to biological and physical characteristics. Gender roles depend on a particular socio-economic, political and cultural context, and are affected by other factors, including age, race, class and ethnicity. Gender roles are learned and

Box 3: Governments Come Together to Fight HIV/AIDS in the Caribbean

A coalition to fight HIV/AIDS in the Caribbean was launched in February 2001 at the CARICOM Heads of Government meeting in Barbados. The region has the highest prevalence of HIV/AIDS outside sub-Saharan Africa. In a population of just over 6 million, an estimated 420,000 people are infected, and AIDS is a major cause of death for the 15–44 age group in several countries.

The new Caribbean Regional Strategic Plan of Action for HIV/AIDS is designed to give governments the tools to intervene quickly to prevent the spread of the disease, with programmes focused on high-risk groups as well as treatment for those living with AIDS. The coalition's goal is to reduce the number of new HIV infections, provide care for people already infected, reduce AIDS-related discrimination and increase the ability of communities, NGOs and others to respond to the epidemic.

Specific targets include cutting HIV transmission from mother to child by 50 per cent by 2003 and reducing by 25 per cent HIV/AIDS prevalence among 15- to 24-year-olds by 2005. By 2005, 90 per cent of young people aged 15–24 should have access to information, education and services to help reduce their vulnerability to HIV infection. The Plan of Action takes into account what has and has not worked elsewhere to prevent and contain the AIDS epidemic. In particular, the coalition recognises that the health sector cannot cope with the disease alone and emphasises the need for a broad-based alliance and strong political leadership.

Source: Epstein, 2001

vary widely within and between cultures … [and] can change. Gender roles help to determine women's access to rights, resources and opportunities." (*'Implementation of the Outcome of the Fourth World Conference on Women'*, A/51/322, paras. 7–14).

Women and men do not generally have equal access to resources such as money, information, power and influence.

Included in the construct of gender are the unequal power relations (social, political, economic) between women and men; the stereotyping of women as inferior; and the greater value that is put on men's roles and functions in society (Chinkin, 2001). Women and men do not generally have equal access to resources such as money, information, power and influence. The sexual division of labour means that women do less highly paid and more socially under-valued work. For example, construction and garbage collection, traditionally male jobs, are better paid than traditionally female jobs such as child care, secretarial work and nursing.

What is gender analysis?

Gender analysis is a tool that uses sex and gender as an organising principle or a way of conceptualising information. It helps to bring out and clarify the nature of the social relationships between men and women and their different social realities, life expectations and economic circumstances. In the area of HIV/AIDS, it identifies how these conditions affect women's and men's susceptibility to infection and their access to, and interaction with, treatment and care. Gender analysis provides a framework for analysing and developing policies, programmes and legislation, and for conducting research and data collection. This framework should also recognise that women and men are not all the same and consider factors such as race, ethnicity, level of ability and sexual orientation.

Gender analysis is a systematic process that takes place throughout the course of a given activity. It is thus involved in development, implementation, monitoring and evaluation. It challenges the assumption that everyone is affected in the same way by, for example, policies, programmes and legislation. It probes concepts, arguments and language used, and reveals and makes explicit the underlying assumptions and values. Where these are shown to be biased or discriminatory, gender analysis points the way to more equitable, inclusive options. It thus involves the collection and use of sex-disaggregated data that reveals the roles and responsibilities of women and men. This data is fed into the policy process to enable assessments of how existing and proposed policies and programmes may affect women and men differently and

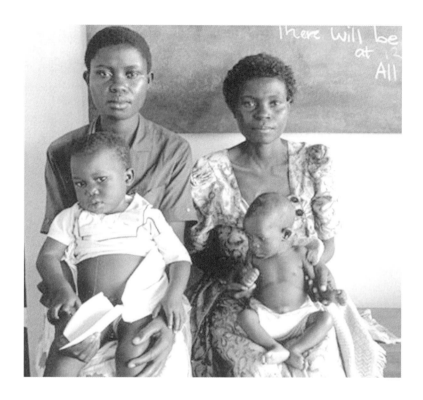

A family visits the AIDS centre in Mbale, Uganda.
Michael Jensen, 2001

unequally. In the area of HIV/AIDS, data needs to be qualitative rather than quantitative if it is to provide useful information about the socially constructed experiences that increase the risk of exposure to infection (Loppie and Gahagan, 2001). Gender analysis also involves assessing how gender roles and gender-inequitable power relations may affect the achievement of a range of development goals, including the goal of gender equality and equity.

Gender analysis is crucial to understanding HIV/AIDS transmission and initiating appropriate programmes of action. It forms the basis for the changes required to create an environment in which women and men can protect themselves and each other. The Commonwealth Secretariat has produced a publication, as part of a programme for the training of health workers in the gender analysis, planning and implementation of health interventions, which includes a valuable section on "Understanding HIV and AIDS: a Global, National and Gender Perspective" (Commonwealth Secretariat, 1999a).

What is gender mainstreaming?

"Mainstreaming a gender perspective is the process of assessing the implications for women and men of any planned action, including legislation, policies or programmes, in any area and at all levels. It is a strategy for making women's as well as men's concerns and experiences an integral dimension in the design, implementation, monitoring and evaluation of policies and programmes in all political, economic and societal spheres so that women and men benefit equally and inequality is not perpetuated. The ultimate goal is to achieve gender equality."

(Agreed conclusions of the UN Economic and Social Council 1997/2)

Gender mainstreaming does not automatically remove the need for women-specific programmes or for projects targeting women. These will often remain necessary to redress particular instances of past discrimination or long-term, systemic discrimination. At the 43rd Session of the UN Commission on the Status of Women (March 1999), member states called for governments "to ensure that the integration of a gender perspective in the mainstream of all government activities is part of a dual and complementary strategy to achieve gender equality. This includes a continuing need for targeted priorities, policies, programmes and positive action measures [for women]" (*Agreed Conclusions on Institutional Mechanisms*). This was endorsed by the UN General Assembly on 1 April 1999. Whenever separate programmes, projects or institutions are set up for women in the context of mainstreaming gender, however, it is vital to ensure that they are accompanied by concrete measures for integration and co-ordination.

Because gender mainstreaming cuts across government sectors and other social partners, it requires strong leadership and organisation. The Commonwealth approach to this is through the Gender Management System (see below).

Why mainstream?

"Gender mainstreaming is based on the recognition that gender equality and equity are: central to national development; a human rights issue that speaks to fairness and social justice for women and men in society; a contributor to good governance in respect of people-oriented, participatory management; and an enabling factor in current efforts at poverty alleviation."

Commonwealth Secretariat, 1999b

Gender mainstreaming is the most efficient and equitable way to use existing resources for combating HIV/AIDS by focusing on the real needs of the whole population. It is required to implement a number of Commonwealth and international mandates. This includes the 1995 Commonwealth Plan of Action on Gender and Development and its Update, in particular the objective of accelerating the achievement of women's empowerment. Through gender mainstreaming, governments will be meeting their commitments to the Nairobi Forward Looking Strategies, agreed to at the Third UN World Conference on Women (1985), and the Beijing Platform for Action (PFA), agreed to at the Fourth UN World Conference on Women (1995). The Beijing PFA urges governments to "promote an active and visible policy of mainstreaming a gender perspective in all programmes and policies" (para. 229).

The need to accelerate the process of mainstreaming a gender perspective was recognised in the Outcome Document adopted at the 23rd Special Session of the General Assembly: 'Women 2000: Gender equality, development and peace for the twenty-first century' (June 2000). Governments are required to: "[d]evelop and use frameworks, guidelines and other practical tools and indicators to accelerate gender mainstreaming, including gender-based research, analytical tools and methodologies, training, case studies, statistics and information" (para. 80).

The Gender Management System

The Commonwealth Secretariat is encouraging the establishment of Gender Management Systems at national and sectoral levels. The Gender Management System is an integrated network of structures, mechanisms and processes put in place in an existing organisational framework in order to guide, plan, monitor and evaluate the process of mainstreaming gender into all areas of an organisation's work. It is intended to advance gender equality and equity through promoting political will; forging a partnership of stakeholders including gov-

Gender mainstreaming is the most efficient and equitable way to use existing resources for combating HIV/AIDS by focusing on the real needs of the whole population.

The goal of a Gender Management System for HIV/AIDS is to ensure gender equality in all government policies, programmes and activities that impact on the epidemic.

ernment, private sector and civil society; building capacity; and sharing good practice. The GMS is described most completely in the *Gender Management System Handbook* (Commonwealth Secretariat, 1999b).

The goal of a Gender Management System for HIV/AIDS is to ensure gender equality in all government policies, programmes and activities that impact on the epidemic. Within the GMS, the design, implementation, monitoring and evaluation of such policies and programmes should not only ensure equality and justice for all regardless of sex and gender, but should also take into account the contributions that can be made by all stakeholders working in the area.

For HIV/AIDS, stakeholders will come not only from the health sector but from a very broad range of ministries and agencies; non-governmental organisations (NGOs), particularly women's organisations; development agencies; the media; trade unions; professional associations; the private sector; and people living with HIV/AIDS. This is because many of the factors that have a major impact on HIV/AIDS lie outside the health sector. For example, within government, decisions about agriculture, finance, education, transport, water and sanitation, employment and social welfare policies all have major and often different effects on women and men. In all these areas, programmes have to deal with such issues as economic power imbalances and social marginalisation. Cultural and traditional attitudes to social roles can also be very important, both in encouraging or condoning practices that increase the vulnerability of men or women and in denying or downgrading the importance of underlying issues such as discrimination.

Objectives

Objectives of the GMS in the context of HIV/AIDS include:

- To promote systematic and consistent gender mainstreaming into HIV/AIDS policies, plans, programmes and activities at all levels.

- To assist state and non-state actors to acquire gender sensitisation, analysis and planning skills necessary for development and implementation of national HIV/AIDS strategies, policies, plans and programmes.

- To strengthen the capacity of National HIV/AIDS Co-ordinating Agencies to direct, advise and co-ordinate national gender mainstreaming efforts in the area of HIV/AIDS.

- To create an enabling gender-inclusive environment in the fight against HIV/AIDS and address the differential impact of the pandemic on women and men at all levels.

The enabling environment

There are a number of interrelated factors that determine the degree to which the environment in which the GMS is being set up does, or does not, enable effective gender mainstreaming. The enabling environment includes the following:

- political and administrative will and commitment at the highest level to gender equality and equity;

- willingness of those stakeholders and implementers who have never been exposed to issues related to gender to acquire knowledge and skills in gender awareness, and gender analysis and planning;

- a legislative and constitutional framework that is conducive to advancing gender equality;

- a 'critical mass' of women in decision-making bodies;

- adequate human and financial resources; and

- an active civil society.

Structures

Enabling all the key stakeholders to participate effectively in the mainstreaming of gender into governments' policy and programming requires the establishment and/or strengthening of formal institutional arrangements within and outside government. These arrangements can be summarised as follows:

- a **Lead Agency** (possibly a National HIV/AIDS Co-ordinating Committee) which initiates and strengthens the GMS institutional arrangements, provides overall co-ordination and monitoring and carries out advocacy, communications, media relations and reporting;

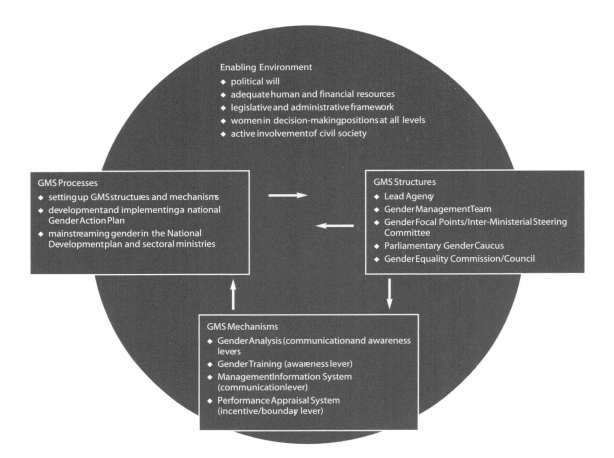

Enabling Environment
- political will
- adequate human and financial resources
- legislative and administrative framework
- women in decision-making positions at all levels
- active involvement of civil society

GMS Processes
- setting up GMS structures and mechanisms
- development and implementing a national Gender Action Plan
- mainstreaming gender in the National Development plan and sectoral ministries

GMS Structures
- Lead Agency
- Gender Management Team
- Gender Focal Points/Inter-Ministerial Steering Committee
- Parliamentary Gender Caucus
- Gender Equality Commission/Council

GMS Mechanisms
- Gender Analysis (communication and awareness levers
- Gender Training (awareness lever)
- Management Information System (communication lever)
- Performance Appraisal System (incentive/boundary lever)

Figure 1: The Gender Management System

- a **Gender Management Team** (consisting of representatives from the Lead Agency, key government ministries and civil society) which provides leadership for the implementation of the GMS; defines broad operational policies, indicators of effectiveness and timeframes for implementation; and co-ordinates and monitors the system's performance;

- an **Inter-Ministerial Steering Committee** whose members are representatives of the Lead Agency and the Gender Focal Points (see below) of all government ministries, and which ensures that gender mainstreaming in government policy, planning and programmes in all sectors is effected and that strong linkages are established between ministries;

- **Gender Focal Points** (senior administrative and technical staff in all government ministries), who identify gender concerns, co-ordinate gender activities (e.g., training); promote gender mainstreaming in the planning, implementation and evaluation of all activities in their respective sectors; and sit on the Inter-Ministerial Steering Committee;

- a **Parliamentary Gender Caucus** (consisting of gender-aware, cross-party female and male parliamentarians) which carries out awareness raising, lobbying and promoting the equal participation of women and men in politics and all aspects of national life and brings a gender perspective to bear on parliamentary structures and procedures, legislation and other matters under debate; and

- **representatives of civil society** (a National Gender Equality Commission/Council, academic institutions, NGOs, professional associations, media and other stakeholders), who represent and advocate the interests and perspectives of autonomous associations in government policy-making and implementation processes.

Mechanisms

There are four principal mechanisms for effecting change in an organisation using a GMS:

- **Gender analysis:** This clarifies the status, opportunities, etc. of men and women. It involves the collection and analysis of sex-disaggregated data which reveals how development activities impact differently on women and men and the effect gender roles and responsibilities have on development efforts.

- **Gender training:** Many of the stakeholders in a GMS will require training in such areas as basic gender awareness and sensitisation, gender analysis, gender planning, the use of gender-sensitive indicators, monitoring and evaluation. Training should also include segments on overcoming hostility to gender mainstreaming and may also need to include conflict prevention and resolution and the management of change.

- **Management Information System:** This is the mechanism for gathering the data necessary for gender analysis and sharing and communicating the findings of that analysis, using sex-disaggregated data and gender-sensitive indicators. More than just a library or resource centre, it is the central repository of gender information and the means by which such information is generated by and disseminated to the key stakeholders in the GMS.

- **Performance Appraisal System:** Based on the results of gender analysis, the GMS should establish realisable targets in specific areas. For example, one target might be to reduce vulnerability to HIV/AIDS by ensuring that at least 90 per cent of young men and women have access to prevention methods by 2005 (indicator adopted at ICPD +5, see Appendix 2). On achievement, further targets should be set. The achievement of these targets should be evaluated both at the individual and departmental level through a gender-aware Performance Appraisal System. This should not be separate from whatever system is already in place for appraising the performance of employees; rather the present system should be reviewed to ensure that it is gender-sensitive. The Performance Appraisal System should also take into account the level of gender sensitivity and skills of individuals (for example, as acquired through gender training or field experience).

2. A Gender Analysis of HIV/AIDS

Overview

Crucial to understanding HIV/AIDS transmission and initiating appropriate programmes of action is an understanding of the socially constructed aspects of relations between women and men that underpin individual behaviour, as well as the gender-based rules, norms and laws governing the broader social and institutional context.

In most societies, gender relations are characterised by an unequal balance of power between men and women, with women having fewer legal rights and less access to education, health services, training, income-generating activities and property. This situation affects both their access to information about HIV/AIDS and the steps that they can take to prevent its transmission. Globally, it is estimated that 90 per cent of all cases of infection now occur through vaginal intercourse (UNIFEM, 2001) and 48 per cent of those newly infected in 2001 were women (55 per cent in sub-Saharan Africa) (UNAIDS/WHO, 2001).

Beyond the statistics of sex-based differences in infection rates, there are profound differences in the underlying causes and consequences of HIV/AIDS infections in women and men. These reflect differences not only in biology but also in sexual behaviour, social attitudes and pressures, economic power and vulnerability. Gender analysis can help researchers and policy-makers understand how fundamental cultural norms of masculinity and femininity influence sexual knowledge and behaviours. It can also identify the changes required to create an environment in which women and men can protect themselves and each other.

HIV/AIDS and Men

While the HIV infection rates of women are fast catching up,

. . . many societies subscribe to the idea that women seduce men into having sex and that men cannot resist because their sexual needs are so strong.

infection rates in men still outnumber those in women in every region except sub-Saharan Africa. Young men are more at risk than older ones: about one in four people with HIV are young men under the age of 25.

Why men are at risk

Through socialisation, both men and women are subject to ideas about what is normal behaviour for women and men; what are 'typical' feminine and masculine characteristics; and how women and men should behave in particular situations. Part of the reason for the high level of HIV/AIDS among men is that many societies subscribe to the idea that women seduce men into having sex and that men cannot resist because their sexual needs are so strong (KIT/SAfAIDS/WHO, 1995). Such beliefs are an obstacle to HIV/AIDS prevention because they absolve men from taking responsibility for their sexual behaviour. As a result of these beliefs, men may be excused for not using condoms or for 'normal masculine behaviour' such as coercing women into intercourse (UNFPA, 2000a). Male condoms are the primary means of preventing HIV transmission during sexual intercourse and men are usually in control of whether this form of protection is used or not. The belief that condoms reduce male pleasure or a concern that their use might indicate infidelity may restrict male usage.

Another problem is the societal expectation that men are knowledgeable about sex. This can make them uncomfortable about admitting that they do not know, limiting their access to information (UNAIDS, 2001a). The cultural beliefs and expectations that make men the ones responsible for deciding when, where and how sex will take place heighten not only women's but men's own vulnerability to HIV and STIs.

All over the world, men tend to have more sexual partners than women, including more extramarital partners. Many societies condone men in having multiple sexual relationships in spite of the clear risks of infection that these pose to their spouse and to their children – and of course to themselves. Male migration and mobility, common in many developing countries where men are forced by economic factors to leave their village and obtain work elsewhere, reinforce this tendency for men to have sexual relationships outside their

Box 4: The Need for Behavioural Changes in Men

The rapid spread of HIV/AIDS among women can only be slowed if concrete changes are brought about in the sexual behaviour of men.

- A study of female youth in South Africa showed that 71 per cent had experienced sex against their will.

- A survey in Tamil Nadu in India showed that 82 per cent of the male STI patients had had sexual intercourse with multiple partners within the last twelve months and only 12 per cent had used a condom.

- A study in India revealed that 90 per cent of the male clients of male sex workers were married.

Source: **Nath, 2001c**

Men may believe that their control of women's lives is an essential element of masculinity.

marriage (Hamblin and Reid, 1991). Predominantly male occupations, such as truck-driving, seafaring and the military, also entail family disruption and create a high demand for commercial sex. When men return home to their households, they re-establish sexual relationships and increase the possibility that HIV/AIDS will be transmitted to rural women (UNIFEM, 2001).

Men may believe that their control of women's lives is an essential element of masculinity. They may become angry or frustrated when they appear to be losing control (UNFPA, 2000a). When gender roles determine that men should provide for their families, those who are unable to do so may respond by becoming dependent on alcohol or inflicting violence on those weaker than themselves, often their partners (UNAIDS, 2001a). Risk and vulnerability are heightened by the link between socialising and alcohol use and by higher frequency among men of drug abuse, including by injection (Nath, 2001b). Men are less likely than women to seek health care or pay attention to their sexual health.

In some parts of the world, men who have sex with men have been disproportionately affected by the HIV epidemic. Contributing factors are multiple sex partners, unprotected

Men need to be involved in prevention and education, and empowered to adopt healthier sexual behaviour.

anal sex and the hidden nature of sexual relations between men in many communities. Risk-taking behaviour may be exacerbated by denial and discrimination, making it difficult to reach them with HIV prevention interventions (Family Health International, 2001b).

Empowering men

Men need to be involved in prevention and education, and empowered to adopt healthier sexual behaviour. This requires a concerted effort by leaders at the highest level, including Presidents, Prime Ministers, parliamentarians, religious leaders, community leaders including chiefs, traditional and spiritual leaders, and leaders of prominent businesses, private organisations and civil society. They need to "speak out as friends, parents, partners and citizens", to affirm their commitment to fight AIDS and to lead by example (UNDPI and UNAIDS, 2001). They should also identify and encourage positive cultural values while discouraging the negative elements preventing men and boys from changing their behaviour.

Since little is known about what men think, and what they might respond successfully to in terms of HIV prevention, it is important to engage them in discussion in order to understand their perceptions, attitudes and practices. The following areas have been suggested as those where research is necessary (Rivers and Aggleton, 1999b):

- Men's beliefs and practices in relation to gender, sex, sexuality and sexual health, especially where the risk of HIV infection is high;

- Sex between men, including an understanding of the meanings attached to male to male sex in the local context;

- Risk-taking behaviour among men, especially among those who work in dangerous and/or isolated environments, since risk-taking appears to be an important part of dominant ideologies of masculinity in a number of societies;

- The kinds of non-stereotypical images and messages that might appeal to men and encourage increased condom use.

As well as health information, education, counselling and

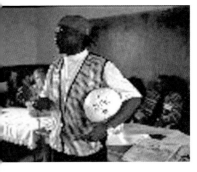

A well-known football player acts as a male role-model as he talks about HIV/AIDS in a school in Kenya
UNAIDS/G. Pirozzi

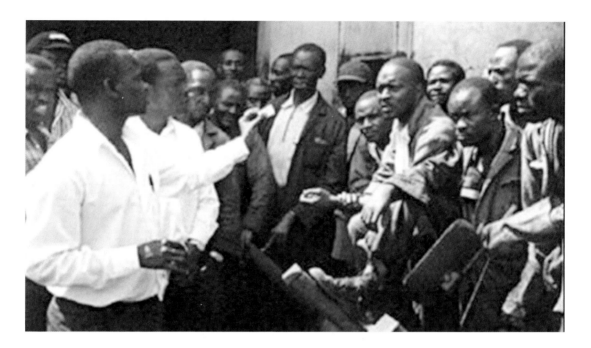

AIDS education work with miners in Southern Africa.
UNAIDS/Jones

services, men should be provided with information about the gender dimensions of HIV/AIDS and the implications of their behaviour for women, families and communities. Men also need information and services for the prevention, early detection and treatment of STIs. Use of the condom is one obvious measure that can help prevent HIV transmission, but programmes at the community level should also promote other healthy options which reduce the spread of HIV, such as mutual fidelity, reduction in number of partners and respect for women's rights (Iwere, 2000). Vaginal microbicides might also prove more acceptable to men than condoms. In a study of 243 men from three sites in South Africa (STI clinics, the general population and universities), more than 80 per cent wanted their partner to be protected against HIV and other STIs. However, the majority also reported a dislike of male condoms and expressed a preference for microbicides. In addition, they were more likely to prefer a vaginal product that prevents HIV and STI transmission and does not act as a contraceptive than one that acts only as a contraceptive (Ramjee et al., 2001).

Gender-based programmes can help men realise that changing the dynamics of male–female relationships so that they are based on collaboration rather than authority can help the

. . . most men, however poor, can choose when, with whom and with what protection, if any, to have sex. Most women cannot.

whole community to minimise the impact of HIV/AIDS. Engaging men and boys as partners will enhance all aspects of sexual and reproductive health, including family planning and child-care (UNFPA, nd).

The risks and needs of men who have sex with men also need to be addressed through, for example, peer education programmes, community-level interventions to reduce risk through safer sex practices, and the creation of 'safe spaces' where they can discuss personal issues and access STI care, counselling and referral services (Family Health International, 2001b).

HIV/AIDS and Women

Globally, almost as many women as men are now dying of HIV/AIDS but the age patterns of infection are significantly different for the two sexes. In many ways, the inequity that women and girls suffer as a result of HIV/AIDS serves as a barometer of their general status in society and the discrimination they encounter in all fields, including health, education and employment.

Lack of control over sex and reproduction

The fact that a man is far more likely than a woman to initiate, dominate and control sexual interactions and reproductive decision-making creates a tremendous barrier to women being able to adopt HIV risk-reducing behaviour. By and large, most men, however poor, can choose when, with whom and with what protection, if any, to have sex. Most women cannot (WHO, 2000b). They are thus often unable to protect themselves against contracting HIV through sexual intercourse, the predominant mode of infection. For many of them, this is not because they have several sexual partners; rather, it is monogamous women who are increasingly at risk of HIV infection because of the sexual behaviour of their steady male partner. An estimated 60–80 per cent of HIV-positive African women have had sexual intercourse solely with their husbands (UNDPI and UNAIDS, 2001). In studies in Papua New Guinea, Jamaica and India women reported that bringing up the issue of condom use, with its inherent implication that one partner or the other has been unfaithful, can result in violence (Gupta, 2002).

Box 5: The Need for Female-Controlled Protection

Women's and girls' vulnerability to HIV infection is four times greater than that of men and boys, and due to many social and economic power imbalances women may not have the power to insist that their sexual partner wear a condom. There is thus a need for a female-controlled form of protection. The female condom is currently the only such method. It is inserted into the vagina and, like the male condom, it provides a barrier to prevent the exchange of body fluids between sexual partners. However, it is difficult for women to use the female condom without their partner's knowledge.

More promise for women-controlled protection may be offered by microbicides which, when inserted into the vagina or rectum, protect against HIV by killing or inactivating the virus. A microbicide could be used without the consent, or even the knowledge, or a woman's partner. There seems to have been some initial reluctance among companies to invest heavily in the development of microbicides since, to be really useful and available to all, they would have to be inexpensive. However, there are currently several candidates heading towards the last phase of human trials within the next two years. Since they are still in the research phase, the efficacy of microbicides is unclear.

Source: UNAIDS, 2001a; Lerner, 2001

A condom, of course, also prevents conception, and a woman's status may depend on her child-bearing ability. Her fertility and her relationship to her husband will often be the source of a woman's social identity (Hamblin and Reid, 1991). Thus, even where women are informed on how to avoid HIV infection, the need for reproduction and their traditionally subordinate role within the family and society, combined with their economic dependence on men, may prevent them from refusing unwanted, and often risky, sexual intercourse.

Worldwide, there are increasingly more poor women than poor men . . .

Growing female poverty

Legal systems and cultural norms in many countries reinforce gender inequality by giving men control over productive resources such as land, through marriage laws that subordinate wives to their husbands and inheritance customs that make males the principal beneficiaries of family property (Tlou, 2001). Worldwide, there are increasingly more poor women than poor men, a phenomenon commonly referred to as the 'feminisation of poverty'. At the same time, women are the sole economic providers in up to one-third of households in the developing world (Gupta, Weiss and Whelan, 1996). Structural adjustment policies imposed by international financial organisations have worsened the situation. Continuing retrenchments and lack of employment opportunities have resulted in women and girls resorting to both direct and indirect commercial sex work as a survival strategy. They may exchange sex for money, food, shelter or other necessities.

Most of this sex is unsafe because women risk losing economic support from men by insisting on safer sex. In a study of low-income women in long-term relationships in Mumbai, India, the women believed that the economic consequences of leaving a relationship that they perceived to be risky were far worse than the health risks of staying in the relationship (Gupta, 2002).

Where substance abuse is also a factor, the means for obtaining clean needles may be traded for other essentials. Trading or sharing needles is a way to reduce drug addiction costs. Risk behaviours and disease potential are predictable under such compromised circumstances (Albertyn, 2000).

Trafficking and sex work

Widespread poverty and the forces of globalisation have also led to an increasing number of women and children being trafficked into prostitution and sexual slavery where they have even less control over their reproductive lives. For example, two million girls between the ages of five and 15 are introduced into the commercial sex market each year (UNFPA, 2000). Rural women may find themselves conned into joining the trade after taking up offers of work in urban areas. These women and children are at extreme risk of disease and death, objectified as a readily attainable and disposable commodity in organised criminal economies.

Stigma and legal status make it difficult for sex workers to access relevant health services. Where sex work is illegal, sex workers may not go for treatment of sexually transmitted infections, increasing the likelihood of HIV infection. They may not seek health care even where sex work is legal, since a diagnosis of an STI may cause the loss of their license and hence their means of support.

A study of sex workers in a southern African industrial community that employs a large number of migrant workers revealed that condom use was extremely rare, despite the fact that most people knew the 'facts' about HIV/AIDS. Women said they lacked the economic power to insist on condom use if paying clients refused to use them. They also lacked the psychological confidence to insist on condom use in a strongly male-dominated culture and noted that if a woman refused sex without a condom, the client would simply find a more willing woman in the shack next door (Mzaidume, Campbell and Williams, 2000).

Some sex workers may actually be more at risk of getting HIV from their intimate partners that from their paying customers. Among commercial sex workers in Glasgow, UK, 90 per cent used condoms with their clients while only 17 per cent used condoms with an intimate partner, even among frequent drug users (UNAIDS, 2001a). Similarly, studies of injection drug use (IDU) in Ontario, Canada found that there was a group of IDU women who have multiple male partners but do not self-identify as being sex workers. While many of them report always using condoms with casual partners, only a very small proportion of these women report always using condoms with their regular partners (Millson et al., 2001).

Lack of information

Because of social pressures and cultural norms, women may also have limited access to information about HIV/AIDS, sexuality and reproductive health. These norms may include an emphasis on women's innocence about sexual matters and girls' virginity. Rural women from South Africa and urban

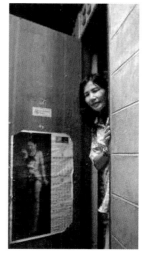

The rate of HIV infection among commercial sex workers in Phayao, Thailand, is about 60 per cent
UNAIDS/Shehzad Noorani

... very little is known about HIV in women as men have formed the vast majority of subjects in studies that form the foundation for the treatment of HIV ...

Box 6: Rising Prostitution in Asia

Prostitution has increased in Asia because of the worsening economic situation in the region. Lack of education and economic opportunities drive young girls and women to large cities in the hope of earning an income. Sometimes they have to prostitute themselves to pay off loans their families had accepted from their future employers. They may also be kidnapped or lured into the sex industry by men whom they trust.

Child prostitution is on the increase, partly because customers are under the mistaken impression that sex with juvenile prostitutes is safer than sex with adult prostitutes. Refugees from political conflicts, sex tourism, local cultural perceptions of manhood, corruption and gender inequality contribute both to the thriving sex industry and the feminisation of poverty. Most sex workers have difficulty protecting themselves against HIV infection because of economic dependency and the threat of physical force. Lesions and injuries in sexual intercourse, especially when they start young, also make them more prone to infections.

Source: Shahabudin, 2000

women from India reported not liking condoms because they feared that if the condom fell off inside the vagina it could get lost and perhaps travel to the throat or another part of the body (Gupta, 2002). Lack of information about their bodies may prevent women from identifying and getting treatment for sexually transmitted infections (STIs), and the overall morbidity and mortality for women from STIs is 4.5 times that of men (UNIFEM, 2001).

At the same time, very little is known about HIV in women as men have formed the vast majority of subjects in studies that form the foundation for the treatment of HIV and opportunistic infections (Nath, 2001a). Women's health is also being "compromised by under-investment in research and product development for female-controlled methods of protection and prevention" (Shahabudin, 2001) and by lack of access to treatment for either HIV/AIDS or the infections associated with it.

Stigma and discrimination

Women may only be tested for HIV/AIDS when they are pregnant, and then only as a measure to protect the unborn child. Since the fathers may not have been tested, the women come to be blamed as the vectors of the epidemic (to partners and children) even though it is almost invariably the husband who passes the HIV infection to his wife. She may be labelled as promiscuous, abused, abandoned or even killed. The man may then seek to marry again, often a younger woman who is believed to be uninfected and therefore safe and who, in turn, will be exposed to HIV.

If her spouse dies, inheritance laws in many countries mean that a woman does not have any rights to the family property and loses her access to land. Alternatively, in many patrilineal African communities, the cultural custom of *levirat* dictates that she has to marry one of her dead husband's brothers in order to continue having access to land and food security. If the husband has died of AIDS, this custom increases the risk of spreading the disease.

In cultures where HIV is seen as a sign of sexual promiscuity,

Workers and patients from The TASO Centre in Kampala, Uganda use drama to provide information about HIV and AIDS.
Michael Jensen, 2001

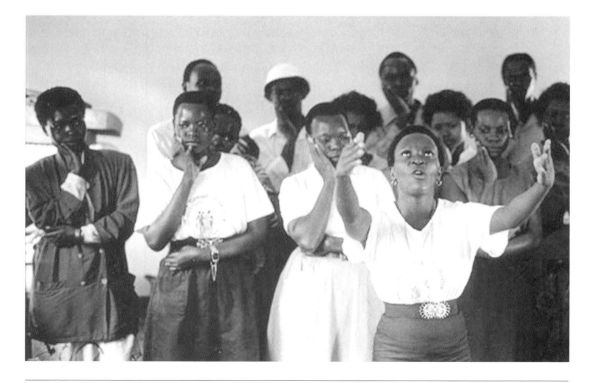

Box 7: HIV/AIDS and Women

- Of the 40 million adults living with HIV/AIDS, 48 per cent – or 17.6 million – are women.

- 48 per cent of adults newly infected with HIV in 2001 were women.

- 49 per cent (1.1 million) of adult AIDS deaths in 2001 were women.

- Since the beginning of the epidemic, over 10 million women have died from HIV/AIDS-related illnesses.

- 55 per cent of all HIV-positive adults in sub-Saharan Africa are women. Teenage girls are infected at a rate 5 or 6 times greater than their male counterparts.

- In one Kenyan study, over one quarter of teenage girls interviewed had had sex before 15, of whom one in 12 was already infected.

- A Zambian study confirmed that less than 25 per cent of women believe that a married woman can refuse to have sex with her husband. Only 11 per cent thought they could ask their husband to use a condom.

- 50 per cent of all HIV-positive adults in the Caribbean are women.

- In Trinidad and Tobago nearly 30 per cent of young girls said they had sex with older men – as a result, HIV rates are five times higher in girls than in boys aged 15–19.

- In the mid-1990s, more than 25 per cent of sex workers in India tested positive for HIV – by 1997 the prevalence rate reached 71 per cent.

Source: UNAIDS *Report on the Global Epidemic,* June 2000; *AIDS Epidemic Update,* December 2000; *Special Session Bulletin 1,* June 2001

HIV-positive women face greater stigmatisation and rejection than men. Those with least access to information or capacity for protection can be excluded from health benefits and treatments and sometimes held to a higher level of responsibility and blame for infection. In Canada, many HIV-positive First Nations women live in secrecy because of the multiple forms of stigma associated with the disease, including being branded 'promiscuous', 'a bad mother' and 'deserving of HIV/AIDS' (Ship and Norton, 2001).

In many countries, men are more likely than women to be admitted to health facilities. Custom and tradition may prevent a woman from travelling alone or receiving medical treatment from a man. Family resources are more likely to be used for buying medication and arranging care for ill males than females (UNDPI and UNAIDS, 2001). Unequal access to health care and the gender gap in medical knowledge contribute to a situation where women in both developed and developing countries have shorter life expectancies than men after a diagnosis of AIDS (UNAIDS, 1997).

. . . women in both developed and developing countries have shorter life expectancies than men after a diagnosis of AIDS.

Women's caregiving role

As social services prove unable to cope with the AIDS epidemic, women are subsidising the public sector by caring for the sick. The societal expectation that women will be the prime or only caregivers to their infected family members creates disproportionate social and economic burdens on them. The cost, time and emotional burden of the disease takes a toll on women that leaves them with little means of protecting themselves or their children from long-term material deprivation.

With the growing infection and death of women from HIV/AIDS, many millions of children will lose their mothers and/or both parents to the epidemic. Many of them will be taken in by grandmothers or other female family members whose care burden is thus increased. The economic costs of care in actual terms by way of medicines and treatment are very high. Families with people living with HIV/AIDS become poor not only because their incomes decline, but because their health expenses increase. Poorer families spend disproportionately more of their income on such expenses. In Kerala, India, it has been estimated that the monthly costs incurred by the family on the treatment of opportunistic infections for an HIV infected child is three times the monthly income of the family (Nath, 2001b). Women head a growing number of poor households.

In rural areas, where women often account for 70 per cent of the agricultural force and 80 per cent of food production, caregiving has been shown to reduce farm output for family consumption and sale (UNAIDS, 2001a). Studies by the Food and Agriculture Organization (FAO) reveal that the pandemic decreases sustainable agricultural production and increases food insecurity. AIDS illnesses and deaths can mean severe labour shortages and loss of productive resources through the sale of livestock to pay for sickness, mourning and funeral expenses (UNFPA, 2000a). This also erodes the family's capacity to provide education and other services to children, and girl children in particular may be taken out of school to help in the home.

Box 8: The Burden of Care

Sixty-six per cent of informal caregivers in Canada are women, representing approximately 14 per cent of all Canadian women over the age of 15. Research among women providing care in rural Nova Scotia found that:

- The majority of the family caregivers reported they were on duty 24 hours a day, seven days a week, caring for people whose ages ranged from four years old to nearly 100.

- Fifteen per cent provided 24-hour care 'with no relief', while 63 per cent received only 'occasional relief'.

- While some had been providing care for only a few months, others had been doing so for as long as 40 years. Many of these caregivers had given up employment in order to provide care; fewer than 25 per cent had paid employment.

- Fifteen per cent of caregivers reported not having enough money to feed all members of the household.

Source: Maritime Centre of Excellence for Women's Health, 1998

Harmful practices

There are also harmful traditional and customary practices that make women and girls more vulnerable, such as early marriage, wife inheritance and wife cleansing. In some parts of the world, women insert external agents into their vaginas, including scouring powders and stones, to dry their vaginal passages in the belief that increased friction is sexually more satisfying to men (Nath, 2001b). This 'dry sex' can cause inflammation and erosion of the vaginal mucosa. Female genital mutilation (FGM) puts girls at risk of HIV if unsterilised instruments are used for several patients in succession. It can also lead to excessive bleeding and tearing when intercourse is attempted (KIT/SAfAIDS/WHO, 1995).

Empowering women

Research done by the International Center for Research on Women (ICRW), USA, has identified six sources of power: information and education; skills; access to services and technologies; access to economic resources; social capital; and the opportunity to have a voice in decision-making at all levels. To empower women (Gupta, 2000b), it is necessary to:

- Educate women and give them the information they need about their bodies and sex;

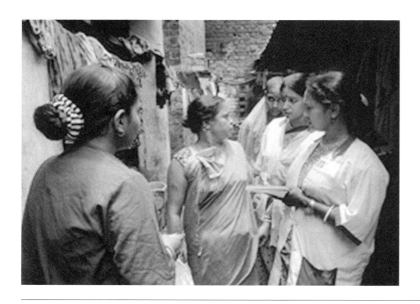

Sex workers in Calcutta, India have organised themselves into a union that provides information on HIV/AIDS.
Michael Jensen, 2001

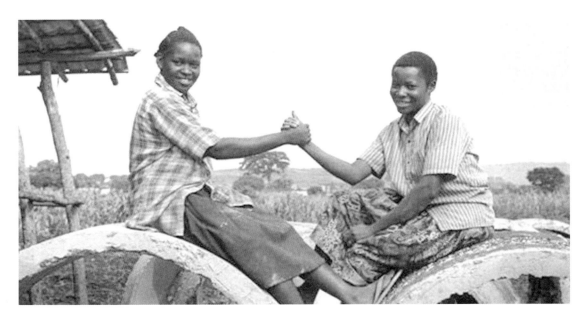

The Masese Women Self Help Project started in a slum area affected by the AIDS epidemic and now sells building materials to projects all over Uganda.
Michael Jensen, 2001

- Provide women with skills-training in communication about sex and how to use a condom, and foster inter-partner communication;

- Improve women's access to economic resources and ensure that they have property and inheritance rights, have access to credit, receive equal pay for equal work, have the financial, marketing and business skills necessary to help their businesses grow, have access to agricultural extension services to ensure the highest yield from their land, have access to formal sector employment, and are protected in the informal sector from exploitation and abuse;

- Ensure that women have access to health services and to HIV and STI prevention technologies that they can control, such as the female condom and microbicides;

- Support the development of an AIDS vaccine that is safe and effective, and accessible to women and young girls;

- Increase social support for women who are struggling to change existing gender norms by giving them opportunities to meet in groups, visibly in communities; by strengthening local women's organisations and providing them with adequate resources; and by promoting sexual and family responsibility among boys and men;

- Move the topic of violence against women from the private sphere to the public sphere, ensuring it is seen as a gross violation of women's rights and not a personal issue;

- Promote women's decision-making at the household, community and national level by supporting their leadership and participation. To give them a voice, they need to be provided with the opportunity to create a group identity separate from that of the family since for many women the family is often the social institution that enforces strict adherence to traditional gender norms.

To reduce the stigma and discrimination faced by women who give birth to children with AIDS, it is important to use the terminology 'parent-to-child transmission (PTCT)', rather than 'mother-to-child transmission (MTCT)'. MTCT focuses attention on the mother as the immediate source of infection, "yet it is well documented that the majority of women have acquired their infection solely through a monogamous relationship with their partner" (Matlin and Spence, 2000). PTCT is a gender-neutral term and hence more appropriate.

Women should be given adequate information about the risks associated with breastfeeding, as well as its benefits, so that they can make an informed decision. HIV passes via breast-feeding to about 1 out of 7 babies born to an HIV-infected woman. However, in many situations where there is a high prevalence of HIV infection, the lack of breastfeeding is also associated with a three-to-five-fold increase in infant mortality (Linkages, 2001). Where there is little or no access to safe water, let alone formula or the money to buy it with, breast-feeding is likely to be the safest method of infant feeding (Machel, 2000).

As women are the majority of HIV/AIDS care providers and deliver most of the unpaid health care within the home, it is important for policy-makers to be aware of how HIV/AIDS health care planning and policy reform affect women and men differently – both as care providers and care recipients. Furthermore, policy-makers and managers need to recognise how health care reform, privatisation and the shift from institutional to home and community-based care affect the lives of women, especially as care-giving affects women's health, productivity and economic security over the life span.

. . . policy-makers and managers need to recognise how health care reform, privatisation and the shift from institutional to home and community-based care affect the lives of women.

Box 9: Empowering Older Women

A pilot project was undertaken in Botswana to strengthen the role of older women in the prevention and control of HIV/AIDS. The empowerment of older women through education, specifically peer education, was seen as important for AIDS prevention. First, older women were able to apply the new knowledge to prevent their own infection with HIV/AIDS, an area that had been neglected due to the incorrect assumption that older women were not sexually active. Second, the women became an important health resource because they learned how to discuss and negotiate with others and educated their families, neighbours and communities about HIV/AIDS prevention and care.

Source: Tlou, 2000

HIV/AIDS and Young People

In many of the heavily affected countries, young people represent the most rapidly growing component of new HIV/AIDS infections, with girls outnumbering boys by a substantial factor. Every minute, six people under the age of 25 become HIV positive. Half of all new HIV infections are in young people aged 15–24. In eight African countries, AIDS is expected to claim the lives of at least a third of today's 15-year-olds. In Botswana, according to the Human Rights Watch website, a 15-year-old boy now has an 85 per cent chance of dying of AIDS.

The reasons for this vulnerability include factors relating to poverty, lack of information, lack of economic and social empowerment, and lack of availability of protective methods. One of the most glaring deficiencies in many countries is the complete absence of adolescent sexual and reproductive health services. Young people often find it difficult to get accurate and practical information on sexual matters from their parents, teachers or health professionals and are forced to rely on inaccurate or incomplete information circulating in peer groups.

Many young women and men tend to ignore risks, falsely

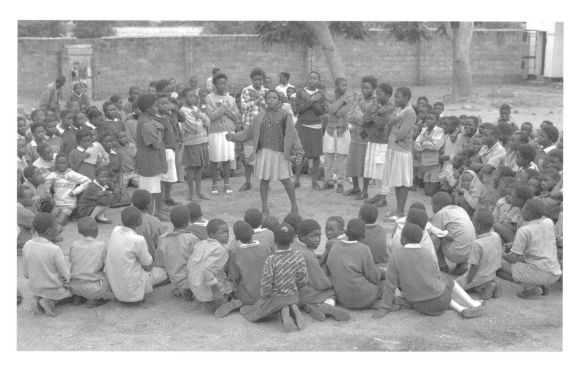

believing that a stable relationship is protection enough. In a number of countries where AIDS is epidemic, nearly half of sexually active girls between the ages of 15–19 believe they face no risk of contracting the disease (UNICEF, 2002). Often, young people will not communicate about sex in early sexual encounters since this maintains "an ambiguity between partners as to whether sex will actually happen" (Kumar, Larkin and Mitchell, 2001) and hence the young man's dignity and the young woman's innocence. Sexual relations may also be unplanned or coerced; young people who are the victims of sexual abuse and exploitation (including incest, rape and forced prostitution) are especially vulnerable to HIV infection (UNDPI and UNAIDS, 2001).

Where sexual and reproductive health services exist, young people find it hard to use them because of lack of money, inconvenient opening times, shame and embarrassment, concerns about privacy and confidentiality, laws that prevent unmarried girls and boys using contraception or require parental consent, and negative and judgmental attitudes of service providers. Young people will avoid seeking STI treatment or contraception if they think that the service providers

Adolescent members of the anti-AIDS club at a primary school in Zambia perform for younger students in the school playground.
UNICEF/HQ96-1233/Giacomo Pirozzi

will not treat them with respect (Commonwealth Secretariat and Healthlink Worldwide, 2001).

An estimated 13.2 million children have been orphaned by AIDS worldwide since the beginning of the epidemic. As well as possibly being infected themselves, they face greater risks of malnutrition, illness, abuse and sexual exploitation than children orphaned by other causes (UNAIDS, 2001b). Marginalised young people (including street children, refugees and migrants) may also be at particular risk because of stigma, their exposure to unprotected sex (in exchange for food, protection or money) and the use of illegal drugs (UNDPI and UNAIDS, 2001). Injecting drug use is rising in young people in some countries, increasing the risk of HIV transmission through sharing contaminated needles and syringes (Commonwealth Secretariat and Healthlink Worldwide, 2001).

Young women

Adolescent girls in a slum in Mumbai, India, listen to a woman discuss ways to refuse unwanted sexual advances as part of a local initiative for girls who are not enrolled in school.
UNICEF/HQ00-0111/
Alexia Lewnes

Young women often have less decision-making power regarding sexuality than adult women, especially because they tend to have older male partners. These men may be better off and able to provide the women with things that they cannot otherwise afford: clothes, cosmetics and even school fees. The relationship may be encouraged by parents in some instances

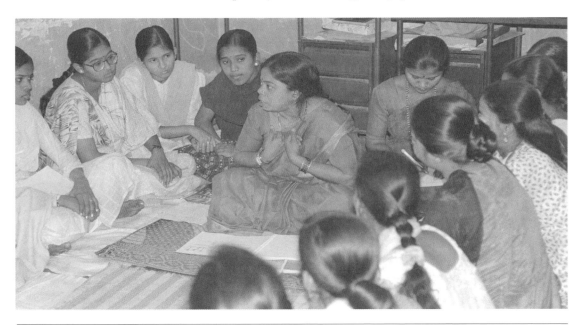

because of financial benefits for the family. These older part-ners can dominate the young women because of their age and gender, and may have had many previous partners and be infected with STIs. Sometimes they actively seek out young girls because they hold the erroneous belief that sex with a virgin can cure a man of infection. Girls also marry at an earlier age than boys.

Young women who show knowledge about sex and repro-duction may be seen as promiscuous and risk getting a "tar-nished sexual reputation" (Kumar, Larkin and Mitchell, 2001). For many young women, discussion around the subject of sex is limited to warnings about its dangers and about the impor-tance of preserving their 'honour' (Rivers and Aggleton, 1999a). Their parents may strictly control their possibilities of accessing services such as contraceptives and condoms (De Bruyn, 2000). Young women are also often expected to be passive, which leaves them with little control over when, where and how sexual activities occur, including the use of condoms (UNAIDS, 2001a).

Biologically, young women are particularly vulnerable because their immature genital tracts may tear during sexual activity, creating a greater risk of HIV transmission. This is especially likely during forced sex. Social expectations may also lead adolescent girls to engage in anal sex to preserve their virginity.

Young men

Like young women, young men are in the phase of establishing their sexual and gender identities, and face various pressures regarding the exercise of their sexuality not only from society at large (parents, religion, the media) but also from their peers (De Bruyn, 2000). Unlike young women, however, young men, are expected to be sexually knowledgeable, which may deter them from seeking information for fear of appearing ignorant. They are also expected to be aggressive and in control of sex-ual relationships. Young men are often encouraged to start having sex from an early age and to have a number of different partners to prove their manhood. There is a lot of pressure on them from their friends and society.

In many countries, a number of young men have their first

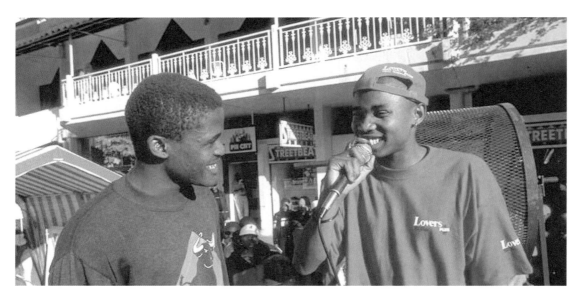

Quiz shows and a radio programme, and condom demo and distribution, attract young people in Gaborone, Botswana.
UNAIDS/G.Pirozzi

sexual experience with other men, sometimes because of the restrictions placed by their culture on socialisation between the sexes (Rivers and Aggleton, 1999a). For a few young men, trading or selling sex to other men may offer a means of survival, and they face many of the same risks as women in a similar position.

While mothers may sometimes take their daughters to clinics for family planning, it is rare for them to take their sons. Boys and young men think that these clinics are for women, and men's sexual health is given a low priority in many countries (Commonwealth Secretariat and Healthlink Worldwide, 2001).

Empowering young people

Engaging young people in addressing HIV/AIDS has become essential; they are the key to controlling the epidemic. Adolescence is the optimum time to develop attitudes and behaviour, and is the critical phase for intervention to ensure that high-risk sexual behaviour patterns do not become entrenched. Behaviour begun in adolescence affects the current and future health of the individual and the population as a whole.

A first step towards effectively protecting adolescents from STIs/HIV is to acknowledge that considerable numbers of

Box 10: Programmes with Young People

Young Men

Working with young men gives them the chance to talk about their feelings and get answers to questions that they cannot risk asking because of expectations that they should know everything. It can also allow them the opportunity to think about what girls and women feel and to practice communication skills. Chogoria Hospital in Kenya conducted a survey of boys coming for circumcision to find out what they knew about HIV and safer sex. There was a lot of misunderstanding and fear, and a strong feeling that after circumcision it was their right to have sex. The hospital introduced an education programme during the week when the boys stay in hospital after the operation which encouraged the young men to consider topics such as becoming a man, sex, STIs/HIV, gender issues and community expectations.

Young Women

In Mumbai, India, World Vision implemented a sex and family life education programme for 76 low-income adolescent girls, the majority of whom were students with additional heavy domestic workloads. The NGO first gained the support of the girls' parents and the wider community through focus group discussions, interviews and the simultaneous implementation of an AIDS awareness programme for the entire community. The programme for the girls ensured that they would be able to attend sessions by providing childcare so that they had time off from caring for their siblings. Highly participatory teaching methods such as story-telling and games focused on helping the girls become more self-confident and able to express their own feelings, opinions and criticisms. Evaluations showed that the girls improved their knowledge about menstruation, reproduction and HIV/AIDS. About 62 per cent had talked to others about HIV/AIDS as well.

Source: Commonwealth Secretariat and Healthlink Worldwide, 2001; UNAIDS, 2001a

Box 11: Seven Principles for AIDS Action among Young People

At the 1995 International Conference on STI/AIDS in Kampala, a group of young Africans from 11 countries put forward a series of seven principles which they saw as essential for effective AIDS action:

- The participation of young people in programme planning, implementation, monitoring and evaluation;

- Provision of youth-friendly services and centres where young people can access information, support and referral;

- Parental involvement in giving better communication, guidance and support to young people;

- Promotion of skills-based education about HIV/AIDS;

- Protection of girls and women against sexual abuse and exploitation, and sensitisation and education of boys and men about their sexuality and behaviour;

- Establishment of networks for young people, including those living with HIV/AIDS, for prevention, protection of human rights and promotion of acceptance by society;

- More commitment and more responsible decision-making by young people themselves about their sexual behaviour and influence on peers.

Source: Matlin and Spence, 2000

young men and women around the world are sexually active. Young women and men need to receive sex education so that they are well-informed about the reproductive process as well as the positive and negative consequences of sex (De Bruyn, 2000). Sexuality education has to de-stigmatise the issue of HIV infection, so that condom use and the risks of unsafe sex can be openly and rationally discussed in the community.

Ideally, education programmes should start before young people become sexually active and should be combined with education about women's rights. By reaching pre-teens and older children, programmes can affect their emerging norms.

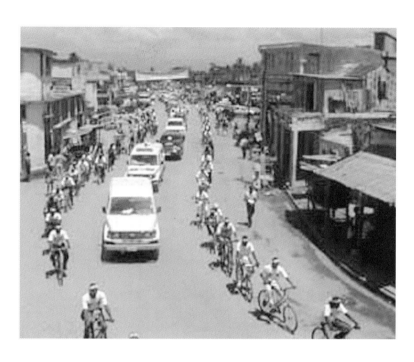

*Participants in the Caravan
of Artists and Youth
Against AIDS in Haiti.*
The Panos Institute/Fritznel Octave

For example, the very young (6- to 10-year-olds) can be exposed to messages about healthy body image, body sovereignty (good touch versus bad touch) and support of people living with HIV/AIDS (Family Health International, 2001a).

Education can also impart negotiation and decision-making skills that young people can use to prevent unwanted sexual relationships and protect themselves from exploitation and violence (UNFPA, nd). Far from sex education promoting promiscuity, numerous studies complied by UNAIDS and its co-sponsors (UNICEF, UNDP, UNFPA, UNDCP, ILO, UNESCO, WHO and the World Bank) have found the opposite to be true. They show that when people have information about sex, they tend to delay sexual intercourse or use condoms, and that it is ignorance that increases their vulnerability to infection (UNAIDS, 2001b).

Discussing cultural taboos around sex, reducing embarrassment and making information and protection available are key factors in achieving better outcomes. Where social and sexual inequities are learned cultural norms, these need to be addressed. It can be counter-productive for educational programmes to ignore the role such norms play in preventing young people from protecting themselves. Calling attention to

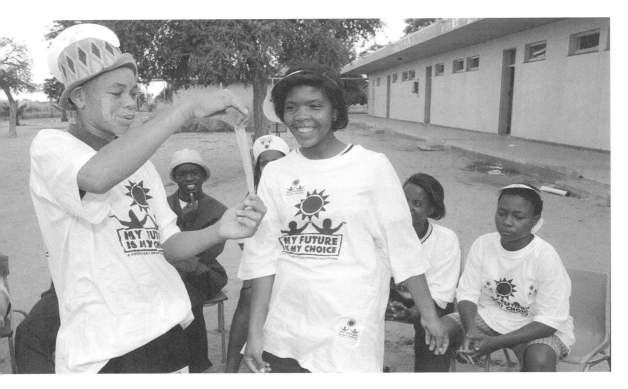

Two secondary school students take part in a role-play about condoms at a meeting of a youth health development programme in Namibia.
UNICEF/HQ00-0103/
Giacomo Pirozzi

them can result in breakthrough behaviours and the gradual acceptance of role changes. Where prevention efforts focus on both young men's and women's responsibilities to prevent disease, the common idea that young women are solely responsible for prevention is gradually weakened. When young women are helped to negotiate personal safety in sexual activity, respect for sexual activity as a mutual decision between equals is reinforced.

Young people are empowered when "they acknowledge that they have or can create choices in life, are aware of the implications of those choices, make an informed decision freely, take action based on that decision and accept responsibility for the consequences of that action" (Commonwealth Secretariat, 1998). They are the best resource for tackling the challenges and problems facing them and should play a central role in AIDS prevention and care programmes. Strategies need to be developed that utilise their energies and expertise, and make them active partners in the design, delivery and evaluation of such programmes. Innovative approaches need to be developed in dealing with different groups of young people, especially those with special needs. Television, radio, street dramas, plays, art, games and the Internet are effectively being utilised to reach young people with messages consistent with their needs. Young people are more likely listen and retain what is being taught when they are also having fun (Family Health International, 2001a).

Since young people respond best to other young people – where they work, study, and play – peer education/promotion/ motivation is a crucial outreach strategy (Family Health International, 2001a). Initiatives such as the Commonwealth Youth Programme's 'Ambassadors for Positive Living' have demonstrated that peer counselling, including that by young people living with HIV/AIDS, can have a powerful effect. These Ambassadors have set up networks of support among HIV-positive youth and meet with their peers in schools, youth groups, churches and military establishments in East and Southern Africa. They have also raised awareness among ministries of youth and health through persistent advocacy and campaigning.

The Role of Gender-based Violence in the Spread of HIV/AIDS

Gender-based violence is a serious problem and an issue both of social justice and human rights and of health and human welfare. It takes many forms and can include physical, emotional or sexual abuse. While both males and females can suffer from gender-based violence, studies show the women, girls and children of both sexes are most often the victims (UNAIDS, 2001a).

One in every three women in the world has been beaten, raped, coerced into sex or physically abused in some way, usually by someone she knows (UNFPA, 2000b). According to the World Bank, gender-based violence accounts for more death and ill health among women aged 15 to 44 worldwide than cancer, traffic injuries and malaria combined (Rose, 2001). The experience of violence, or fear that it might take place, disempowers women in their homes, workplaces and communities and limits their ability to participate in and benefit from initiatives for HIV prevention and AIDS mitigation (Southern African AIDS Training Programme, 2001).

The most pervasive form of gender-based violence is that committed against a woman by her intimate partner.

Domestic violence

The most pervasive form of gender-based violence is that committed against a woman by her intimate partner. Between 10 and 50 per cent of all women worldwide report physical abuse of this kind (WHO, 2000a). Violence between intimate partners is often connected to marital rape, coerced sex or other forms of abuse that lead to HIV risk. A study in Tanzania, for example, showed that women specifically avoided raising the issue of condoms with their husbands for fear of violent retaliation, while fewer than 25 per cent of Zambian women agreed that a woman could refuse to have sex with her husband, even if he was known to be violent, unfaithful or HIV positive (UNAIDS, 2001a). Research amongst HIV-positive African-American women in the USA and poor HIV-positive women in Canada has also found violence to be a central feature of their lives (Albertyn, 2000).

The worldwide prevalence and tolerance of violence against women at individual and systemic levels seriously limits their abilities to protect themselves or their children from sexually transmitted infections. All forms of coerced sex – from violent rape to cultural/economic obligations to have sex when it is not really wanted – increase the risk of microlesions and therefore of STI/HIV infection (WHO, 2000b). Young women are especially vulnerable since their immature genital tract is more likely to tear during sexual activity.

A study of young women in South Africa revealed that 30 per cent reported that their first sexual intercourse was forced, 71 per cent reported having had sex against their will and 11 per cent reported being raped (UNAIDS, 1999). A recent study by Sakshi, an NGO in India, has shown that 60 per cent of the 13–15-year-olds in schools studied had been victims of some kind of sexual abuse, 40 per cent within families, and 25 per cent were victims of serious abuse such as rape (Nath, 2001b). Women later in life are also particularly vulnerable to violence as a result of economic insecurity and, in some societies, diminished social status. Violence against older women can include rape, posing a risk of HIV transmission (UNAIDS, 2001a).

Box 12: Health Canada Initiatives on HIV and Sexual Violence Against Women

Since 1997, Health Canada has funded a series of initiatives on HIV and sexual violence against women. The main objectives of these initiatives are to raise awareness of the links between HIV and violence against women and to provide counsellors and survivors with up-to-date information in this area. The initiatives include:

- a guide for counsellors that addresses the connections between HIV and various forms of violence against women, and related issues such as risk reduction, HIV testing and post-exposure treatment;

- a training manual that provides information on how to plan and implement community training related to HIV and sexual violence;

- a brochure on HIV and sexual assault for survivors, and Asian, Aboriginal and Inuit ethno-cultural adaptations of the brochure.

These are available from the Canadian HIV/AIDS Clearinghouse website at www.clearinghouse.cpha.ca/clearinghouse_e.htm (Toll free phone: 1-877-999-7740, fax: 613-725-1205)

Situations of armed conflict

Gender-based violence is particularly prevalent in armed conflicts, with hundreds of thousands of women raped in wars during the last century. Women and girls make up 75 per cent of the world's 22 million refugees, asylum seekers or internally displaced persons, putting them at particular risk of such violence. Women can be raped by all sides in a conflict. The 10-year-old civil war in Sierra Leone, for example, was characterised by many instances of physical and sexual abuse of women and, in some rural areas, women were forced to give sexual favours to their 'protectors', whether rebels, soldiers or Civil Defence Forces (Forster, 2000).

Military personnel tend to have rates of STIs – which can

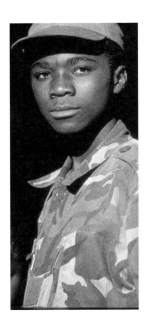

A child soldier in Luena, Angola. Soldiers can be at major risk of acquiring and passing on HIV.
UNAIDS/Chris Sattlberger

increase the risk of HIV – two to five times higher than those of the civilian population even during peacetime. During armed conflict, the rate can increase by 50 times. In Sierra Leone, over 60 per cent of the soldiers tested were reported to be HIV positive (Forster, 2000). Since soldiers are typically young, sexually active men, they are also likely to seek commercial sex (Machel, 2001), increasing the spread of infection.

The social upheaval caused by armed conflict – including loss of local social systems and mass migration – also contributes to the spread of the disease. War breaks up families and communities. It destroys the health services that could identify the diseases associated with HIV/AIDS or screen the blood transfusions that might transmit it, and destroys the education systems that could teach prevention and slow the number of infections (Machel, 2000). It forces women to sell themselves as a means of survival. HIV/AIDS also serves to prolong conflict as it places new strains on health and economic infrastructures and destabilises family and social structures (Kristoffersson, 2000). The links between AIDS and conflict thus run in both directions and reinforce each other, and both are exacerbated by poverty and the gender dimensions of conflict and the pandemic (Machel, 2000).

The UN has declared AIDS to be a security issue because of the potential of conflicts to create the enabling environment for the spread of HIV and other STIs (Forster, 2000). The UN Security Council Resolution on Women, Peace and Security (United Nations, 2000) asks states to incorporate HIV/AIDS awareness training into their national training programmes for military and civilian police personnel, as well as guidelines and materials on the protection, rights and the particular needs of women. It recommends that civilian personnel of peacekeeping operations should receive similar training.

3. A Multisectoral Response to HIV/AIDS

The Need for a Multisectoral and Expanded Response

Introduction

A multisectoral response means involving all sectors of society – governments, business, civil society organisations, communities and people living with HIV/AIDS – at all levels – pan-Commonwealth, national and community – in addressing the causes and impact of the HIV/AIDS epidemic. Such a response requires action to engender political will, leadership and co-ordination, and to develop and sustain new partnerships and ways of working, and to strengthen the capacity of all sectors to make an effective contribution.

Commonwealth Secretariat, 2001

A multisectoral and expanded response to HIV/AIDS is central to current strategies for combating the epidemic. It was agreed to by governments in their Declaration of Commitment at the June 2001 UN General Assembly Special Session on HIV/AIDS (see Appendix 2). This recognised that, since HIV/AIDS is not only a health issue but a development issue that has an impact on every aspect of life, it requires a response from all sectors of society: government, civil society and the private sector.

All government ministries have a key role to play, not just the Ministry of Health. For example, the Ministry of Labour can promote workplace prevention and care programmes, while the Ministry of Education can ensure that AIDS education is taught in schools. Partnerships should be developed to involve collaboration with businesses, non-governmental organisations and communities across different sectors and at various levels.

No policy sector is immune to or unaffected by the impacts of HIV/AIDS and all sectors must commit themselves to plan and make available resources for an integrated response. This must include plans within each sector for its own activities that will contribute to the national fight against AIDS. These include an analysis of the factors contributing to the spread of HIV/AIDS, the impact of the disease on its workforce and products and the consequences for both the sector and the community. Practical short-term and long-term interventions must also be developed to protect the sector's workers, to cope with the skills shortages that will arise and to mitigate the adverse effects on society.

Box 13: A Framework for Assessing the Impact of HIV/AIDS on a Sector

- Define the sector and its activities;

- Identify the risk factors for HIV/AIDS for both women and men;

- Assess the impact of HIV/AIDS on the sector;

- Assess sectoral strategies to maintain the workforce

  - Training

  - Multi-skilling

  - Importation of labour;

- Assess sectoral response to HIV/AIDS

  - HIV/AIDS workplace policy and programme

  - Access to prevention and treatment

  - Family support

  - Non-discriminatory practices.

Source: HIV/AIDS Fact Sheets, Commonwealth Secretariat

The experience of UNAIDS has shown that such an expanded response must also include the following elements (UNAIDS, 2001b):

- constant, visible examples that promote openness about HIV/AIDS and defuse the associated stigma and discrimination;

- coherent national strategies and plans that draw a wide range of actors from the state and civil society;

- social policy reforms that reduce people's vulnerability to HIV infection;

- strategies grounded in communities' activities and mobilisation (these communities must also be enabled to rise to the challenge);

- the involvement of people living with HIV/AIDS (PLHA);

- broad and equitable access to prevention and care, as well as the realisation that these dimensions are inseparable;

- the translation of lessons learned back into practice; and

- adequate resources deployed nationally and globally against the epidemic.

Among the lessons learned are that different partners bring different strengths and that leadership needs to be exercised at all levels and by all sectors. Sectors need to be involved on the basis of their comparative advantage and potential contribution to the issue concerned. To meet the needs of adolescents, for example, a group of NGOs, the District Health Management Team and UNICEF formed an Adolescent Health Task Force in Zambia that established Youth Friendly Health Services. They mobilised political commitment, trained peer educators and established links between NGOs, clinics and young people.

In all areas, programmes should deal with issues of economic power imbalances, migrations, economic and social marginalisation, development of community responses, participation and capacity building for sustainability. Mechanisms have to be developed to involve the private sector, PLHA, religious groups, community leaders, the media and other stakeholders. Experiences of partnership development and best practices in multisectoral responses need to be shared. The role of education should be recognised as a key channel through which knowledge and skills essential for individual, community and national survival can be imparted.

Box 14: Objectives of a Multisectoral Approach

- To link HIV/AIDS to all poverty reduction strategies and other actions aimed at improving quality of life.

- To recognise that people living with HIV/AIDS (PLHA) must be central to responses and that their participation and empowerment to enable them to take effective action themselves and with others is essential to success.

- To promote political will and mobilise action to break the silence about HIV/AIDS, reduce discrimination and stigma, protect the human rights of PLHA, provide effective programmes to prevent, treat, care for and mitigate the impact of HIV/AIDS, and mobilise and make available resources for civil society organisations engaged in prevention and care.

- To pay particular attention to the specific needs of adolescents and young people, especially girls, in order to prevent them from becoming infected.

- To address the needs of vulnerable and disadvantaged groups, such as the majority of women and girls in developing countries, those living in poverty, street children, the disabled, migrants, refugees, sex workers, people in detention, those living in conflict zones, injecting drug users, and men who have sex with men.

- To ensure that the needs of those caring for PLHA are taken into account.

- To promote policies that enable communities to take effective action themselves and with others to prevent HIV infection and to improve the quality of life of PLHA.

- To facilitate partnerships among all agencies at local, national and international levels, recognising the important roles that civil society and the private sector can play.

- To expand efforts and improve methods for prevention, treatment and care. This includes providing access to

affordable drugs that alleviate the symptoms and opportunistic infections associated with HIV and reduce parent-to-child transmission, and vigorously pursuing innovative measures including vaccines, microbicides and traditional and complementary therapies that are appropriate and affordable for those living in developing countries.

Source: **Commonwealth Secretariat, 2001**

Key aspects of a multisectoral response

A background paper prepared for a Commonwealth Think Tank meeting on 'A Multisectoral Response to Combating HIV/AIDS in Commonwealth Countries' held in July 2001 identified the following key aspects of a multisectoral response (Commonwealth Secretariat, 2001):

- Considering HIV/AIDS and its implications in all areas of policy-making;

- Involving all sectors in developing a framework to respond to the epidemic, at international, regional, national, district and community levels;

- Identifying the comparative advantages and roles of each sector in implementing the response, and where sectors need to take action together and individually;

- Encouraging each sector to consider how it is affected by and affects the epidemic, and developing sectoral plans of action;

- Developing partnerships within government between ministries responsible for different sectors, and between the public sector, private sector and civil society.

The pattern of HIV transmission and the stage of the epidemic are different in each country, depending on the underlying social, economic, political and cultural context. A national consensus and a common vision of what needs to be done in that particular country has, therefore, to be developed. The Gender Management System is flexible enough to be adapted

Table 3: Framework for a Multisectoral Response at National Level

	Government	Business	Civil Society Organisations
Actors	Heads of State Government Ministers and MPs Political leaders at central and local government levels Civil servants at central and local government levels	Chief Executives Managing Directors Boards of Directors Managers	University and educational leaders Religious and community leaders including traditional and spiritual healers NGOs Trades union leaders Leaders of professional associations Women's and youth leaders Traditional political leaders PLHA, people affected, orphans
Sectors	Health Education Social Welfare Water and Sanitation Finance Gender/Women Labour Transport Industry, Commerce, Agriculture Defence Culture and National Heritage Youth Home Affairs Public Service Information and Broadcasting	Insurance Banking Beverages Human Resource Development Construction Tourism, Pharmaceuticals Mining MFI, medium and small enterprises	NGOs and charitable organisations Women's organisations and groups Professional associations Religious organisations Traditional, community and cultural leaders PLHA Media Traditional healers
Resources	Human resources Physical infrastructure Funds	Human resources Physical infrastructure Funds	Human resources, families and extended families

Source: Commonwealth Secretariat, 2002.

to the issue of HIV/AIDS and to the distinctive national context (see Chapter 1 and below).

The response must be dynamic and react to the epidemic as it evolves. Strong and creative leadership is called for and political will at the highest level is critical. The government must take the lead in fostering a supportive environment and providing a framework for action. The framework should take account of the response's need to work both horizontally (with government, business and civil society organisations) and vertically (at international, national and community levels).

It is critical that the approach integrates prevention and care. With regard to prevention, focusing on individual behav-

Table 4: Framework for a Multisectoral Response at Community Level

	Government	Business	Civil Society Organisations
Actors	Local government officers and chiefs Bureaucrats Local chiefs and community leaders Social welfare officers Politicians Health workers Agricultural, forestry, and veterinary extension workers Other development workers	Commercial farmers Traders Retailers and food sellers Pharmacies Manufacturers Media	PLHA Religious and community leaders Teachers Parents and grandparents NGOs, CBOs and ASOs Women's organisations and groups Trades unions Vulnerable groups e.g. IDUs, SWs Community media Associations e.g. women, youth, poverty action Subsistence farmers Formal and informal sector workers Community volunteers Traditional political leaders Traditional healers
Sectors	Transport Industry, trade and mining Education Health Legal and justice Community Development Culture Youth Agriculture Information Traditional political leaders' associations	Transport Industry, trade, commerce and mining Retailing	Prominent individuals e.g. sportspersons, musicians Professional associations Cultural organisations Religious organisations
Resources*	Primary health centres, schools and other government facilities Funds	Volunteers and mentors Funds Skills AIDS aware workforce Commodities e.g. condoms, drugs	People Trained professionals Aware media Community groups e.g. handicraft, income generation Human spirit, inner strength Families

*International donors

Source: Commonwealth Secretariat, 2002.

iour change is insufficient since poor health (including malnutrition, untreated STIs, malaria and other parasites), gender, poverty and other factors also play an important role in vulnerability and susceptibility to HIV. The poorest and most vulnerable groups, including women and young people, need to be seen as resources and positive contributors, and not just victims.

Box 15: The Effectiveness of a Multisectoral Approach: Uganda

Uganda had runaway HIV infection rates until the early 1990s, the highest prevalence in the world, but has used a multisectoral approach to curb them. In addition to widespread public information campaigns, Ugandan officials have promoted the participation of state, local, non-governmental and community-based agencies in the fight against the epidemic. In recognition that the disease has consequences far beyond the health sector, the Uganda AIDS Commission was established in 1992 under the Office of the President. The government emphasises the collective responsibility of individuals, community groups, different levels of government and other agencies for the prevention of HIV infection, mitigation of the impact of the epidemic on individuals and communities and provision of care and compassion. A society-wide movement has been mobilised to empower people to protect themselves against infection and to fight stigma and discrimination against people living with HIV/AIDS.

HIV/AIDS has been mainstreamed in the budget with the Poverty Eradication Action Programme in order to increase the capacity of local authorities to deal with the disease. Civil society and the private sector have also become involved. For example, the business community has established a Uganda Business Council on HIV/AIDS to support the promotion of prevention and care programmes in the workplace. The government has also stepped up its advocacy using the media and performing arts, creating high levels of awareness about the disease among the population.

The HIV adult prevalence rate is estimated to have dropped from over 30 per cent in 1993 to 14 per cent in 1995 to below 8 per cent in 2000. Rates of infection among girls aged 13–19 dropped from 4.4 per cent in 1989–1990 to 1.4 per cent in 1996–1997. Reports also indicate that in the capital city of Kampala, the number of HIV-positive pregnant women – which peaked at three in ten in the early 1990s – has also fallen sharply.

Source: UNAIDS, 2001a; Shames, 2000; UNDP, 2001

Mainstreaming gender into the multisectoral response

It is vital that in developing and applying this multisectoral response the concept of gender is included at every stage. An understanding of the gender issues and dimensions of HIV/AIDS must be central to the analysis of causes and contributory factors as well as to the planning and execution of responses, whether these are aimed at preventing transmission or mitigating the impacts of the disease. In short, gender must be 'mainstreamed' into the multisectoral response to HIV/AIDS.

The implications of this statement are profound, because gender mainstreaming calls for skills in gender-based understanding, analysis and planning; the capacity to collect and interpret sex-disaggregated data; a commitment by government to take action to achieve gender equality; and the availability of human, technical and financial resources. Some or all of these may be in short supply in countries where they are needed most. Gender concerns have not been adequately addressed in existing multisectoral responses to HIV/AIDS, partly because there is a skills gap in gender sensitisation and analysis among senior policy makers, middle level professionals and others involved in the design and implementation of these responses. The following components are therefore critical for effective gender mainstreaming in this area:

- Building capacity for training in gender sensitisation and analysis for all key professionals and workers at national and local levels (including developing locally relevant training materials, training of trainers, and allocating time and resources);

- Establishing system-wide processes in each sector to oversee programme development, implementation, monitoring and evaluation, taking into account women's and men's needs, interests and contributions;

- Enhancing capacities for the collection, analysis and use of sex-disaggregated data.

Government analysts and decision-makers need to factor in gender indicators as they prepare national HIV/AIDS policy guidelines that are culturally appropriate. Broad-based national frameworks and methodologies for practical gender

An understanding of the gender issues and dimensions of HIV/AIDS must be central to the analysis of causes and contributory factors . . .

A training session for peer educators at the NGO Kindlimuka, an association of people living with HIV/AIDS in Mozambique.
UNICEF/HQ01-0168/Giacomo Pirozzi

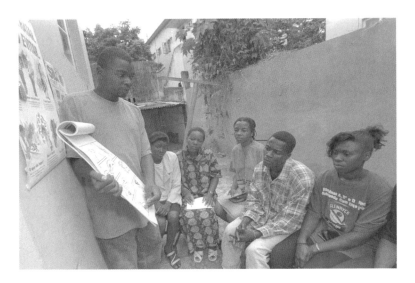

mainstreaming programmes, including gender equality and health indicators, need to be tailored to specific cultural contexts since these affect sexual roles, behaviour, attitudes and power relationships.

In promoting 'safer sex' as a public health message, policy-makers must also take into consideration the different impact of this message on men and women. Many of the strategies to prevent the spread of HIV/AIDS have focused on promoting condom use, reducing the number of sexual partners and treating STIs. However, these fail to address the social, economic and power relations between men and women (see Chapter 2). A policy and programme that attempts to reach vulnerable populations in this limited way may miss the opportunity for key and strategic investments. Targeted HIV/AIDS prevention strategies are more likely to both reach and influence high-risk populations.

Gender not only impacts on preventive strategies to reduce the sexual transmission of HIV/AIDS but also affects compliance with treatment protocols. Both short- and long-term gender-sensitive strategies need to be developed from the community to the national level. Short-term strategies might focus on people's immediate needs, such as information (for both literate and illiterate populations), support for home-based care and access to treatment for STIs. More long-term strategies need to address the underlying social and cultural structures that sustain gender inequality (UNFPA, 2000a).

Box 16: Examples of Multisectoral Responses at Different Levels

International

The International Partnership on AIDS in Africa (IPAA) involves African governments, UNAIDS and its co-sponsors (UNICEF, UNDP, UNFPA, UNCDP, UNESCO, WHO and the World Bank), bilateral donor agencies, the private sector and civil society in an initiative to slow the spread of HIV/AIDS and mitigate the impact of the epidemic. IPPA focuses on: developing a framework for collaboration; raising political support; mobilising resources; producing National Strategic Plans; establishing and strengthening National AIDS Councils or similar co-ordinating bodies; decentralising national responses to regional, provincial and district levels; and scaling up specific programmes such as voluntary counselling and testing, prevention of parent-to-child transmission and care and support for people living with HIV/AIDS (PLHA).

Regional

The Southern African Development Community (SADC) held a regional conference in Malawi in 1996 which brought together policy-makers and other key actors from the employment, mining, tourism, migration and education sectors and which formulated a number of actions in each sector. In 2000, SADC issued an HIV/AIDS Strategic Framework and Programme 2000–2004 in an effort to decentralise the responses of the various sectors to apply their areas of highest comparative advantage to address the pandemic. This was not gender-sensitive, however, and a process is currently underway to engender it. Partners in this process include the UN Economic Commission for Africa Sub-Regional Development Centre in Lusaka, the SADC Gender Unit, UNIFEM, SADC Health Co-ordinating Unit, the Commonwealth Secretariat, NGOs and national machineries.

National

Botswana is mainstreaming HIV/AIDS into the plans of all government ministries, NGO and private sector partners.

(*continued on page 62*)

Box 16 (*continued*)

For example, the Division of Social Welfare is responsible for administering a food basket programme for PLHA.

Provincial/ district
In the Eastern Cape province of South Africa, the Bamisanani programme, involving the Employment Bureau of South Africa, Mineworkers Development Agency and Planned Parenthood Association of South Africa, provides services to meet the social, economic and health care needs of PLHA and affected and vulnerable populations.

Source: Commonwealth Secretariat, 2001; Lomayani, 2002

Using a GMS approach

The establishment of a national GMS to tackle HIV/AIDS will involve a number of key stages:

- Sensitisation of the key stakeholders (government ministries and agencies, NGOs, the private sector and people living with HIV/AIDS) to the needs and opportunities;

- Detailed planning of a system which meets national requirements and which is set in the context of local economic and cultural factors;

- Generation of political commitment leading to effective political action;

- Sustained efforts at all levels to maintain momentum and ensure continued responsiveness and relevance of the GMS.

Application of the GMS to HIV/AIDS is carried out with a number of assumptions related to governments' commitments (Commonwealth Secretariat, 2002). These include that governments:

- Will adopt a multisectoral approach to HIV/AIDS, if they have not already done so;

- Have an obligation to promote gender equality and human

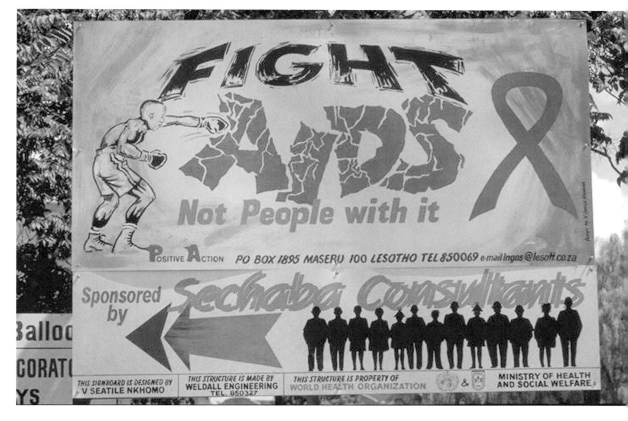

Billboard on AIDS prevention produced by an NGO called Positive Action based in Maseru, Lesotho.
UNAIDS/G. Pirozzi

rights as enshrined in international and regional human rights standards and other mandates;

- Can put in place a constitutional and legislative framework to promote gender equality and protect the human rights of women, prevent gender-based violence, and protect the rights of people living with HIV/AIDS;

- Have the political will at the highest level to do all that is necessary to promote gender equality and address discrimination against women in all HIV/AIDS interventions;

- Will be able to commit the human, institutional and financial resources necessary for effective gender mainstreaming;

- Will increase the effectiveness of current strategies and control the HIV/AIDS pandemic by targeting women and girls;

- Will promote multi-disciplinary efforts and the implicit interdepartmental collaboration and co-ordination within and outside government structures. The GMS in HIV/AIDS depends on joint and co-ordinated effort at different levels of government, civil society and the private sector;

● Will increase the participation of women in the decision-making process in the political, public and private sector, which is fundamental to combating HIV/AIDS.

The UN Secretary-General, in his report on the thematic issues addressed by the 43rd session of the Commission on the Status of Women, emphasised the effectiveness of the Gender Management System as a tool that "take[s] into account the need for sensitisation and training of actors at all levels" (United Nations, 1999).

It is also important to take stock of national and local realities and needs. Country reports on gender and development prepared by government will be useful in providing the context within which the GMS will operate. These include, for example, reports for the UN 4th World Conference on Women (Beijing 1995) or to the Committee on the Elimination of Discrimination against Women (CEDAW); reports prepared by NGOs; other national and regional reports and reports of relevant international meetings; and National Development Plans and national policies on women.

Examples of HIV/AIDS Issues and Responses by Sector

Agriculture

It is likely that the AIDS epidemic will cause a major agricultural labour shortage in many countries, with 7 million agricultural workers already lost and at least 16 million more who could die before 2020 in sub-Saharan Africa. An FAO study in Namibia showed that for all types of households in farming communities AIDS deaths also meant the "loss of productive resources through the sale of livestock to pay for sickness, mourning and funeral expenses, as well as a sharp decline in crop production" (UNFPA, 2000a).

Sickness also contributes to the scarcity of labour because of both the incapacity of workers and the time others have to devote to looking after them. If a family member is sick with

Box 17: Why Use the Gender Management System?

Applying the GMS principles to the area of HIV/AIDS will bridge the gender mainstreaming gaps that exist in current strategies and interventions. The purpose is to:

- Promote commitment, programme ownership and co-ordination at all levels for an integrated multisectoral approach to the control and prevention of HIV/AIDS;

- Increase understanding of the impact of culture, gender and social relations to the spread and prevention of HIV/AIDS;

- Increase gender awareness and analysis skills required for designing gender-responsive policies and programmes;

- Respond directly to the needs of women, men and young people infected and affected by HIV/AIDS;

- Take appropriate action, particularly with regard to men's contribution to controlling the pandemic;

- Change societal values, attitudes and behavioural patterns that fuel the pandemic;

- Modify existing structures and systems (such as legal, educational, economic) which support the existing power imbalance between women and men in society;

- Identify stakeholders and possible partners at all levels;

- Share experiences and resources and exchange information, ultimately leading to better co-ordination and collaboration;

- Prepare a plan of action with concrete activities at all levels in order to effectively target women and men, as well as girls and boys, in the fight against HIV/AIDS;

- Build capacities within relevant government and non-government sectors for greater efficiency.

Source: Commonwealth Secretariat, 2002

AIDS, women may be unable to perform such labour-intensive and significant tasks as watering, planting, fertilising, weeding, harvesting and marketing. In many rural areas, women account for 70 per cent of the agricultural labour force and 80 per cent of food production (UNAIDS, 2001a). With lost labour, nutritious leafy crops and fruits may be replaced by starchy root crops, while the sale of livestock means less milk, eggs and meat. Chronic food insecurity can result, together with high levels of malnutrition and micronutrient deficiencies which further compromise immune systems (Loewenson and Whiteside, 2001).

In addition, the deaths of farmers, extension workers and teachers from AIDS can undermine the transmission of knowledge and know-how and the local capacity to absorb technology transfers. A study in Kenya has shown that only 7 per cent of farming households headed by orphans have adequate knowledge of agricultural production (UNDPI and UNAIDS, 2001). Since men have more access to productive resources such as land, credit and technology, their widows may be left without such access and these women's livelihood may be threatened. HIV/AIDS is also reducing investment in irrigation, soil enhancement and other capital improvements.

Policy/Action/Intervention

- Initiate outreach on HIV/AIDS to rural communities.

- Support poverty relief and food security programmes.

- Ensure that rural development and food security policies take into account the different realities of women and men as well as the impact of HIV/AIDS.

- Ensure women's access to productive resources, including land, credit and other agricultural facilities.

- Facilitate interventions to support rural families, including those catering for orphans and those that support the empowerment of rural women.

- Involve agricultural extension officers in HIV/AIDS activities.

- Encourage commercial farmers' organisations to develop responses to HIV/AIDS.

- Integrate awareness raising, e.g., through the use of drama, into agricultural shows.

Box 18: Responding to HIV/AIDS and Agriculture (A Global Initiative)

The Global Initiative on HIV/AIDS, Agriculture and Food Security (GIAAFS) is intended to help mitigate and prevent the spread and negative impact of HIV/AIDS on agriculture, food and nutrition security. It is facilitated by the Consultative Group on International Agricultural Research (CGIAR), a network of 16 international agricultural research centres with more than 50 members worldwide. The initiative stresses the need for research to understand and link the HIV/AIDS pandemic with rural, peri-urban and urban livelihoods systems, agricultural land use, food and nutrition security and social structures. The aim is to make public and private investments in primary rural industries more attractive; improve rural livelihoods; reduce rural to urban migration; and improve human nutrition and immune responses. The participation of women is seen to be especially important, because of the critical role they play in household food security and the wellbeing of children.

Source: Abamu, 2002

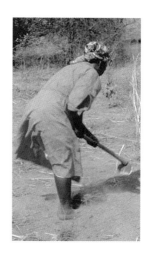

A woman prepares her fields for planting in Zimbabwe.
UNAIDS/L. Alyanak

- Encourage men to participate in foodcrop production, especially managing home gardens for growing nutrient supplements for those infected with HIV/AIDS.

Education

In many countries with high HIV/AIDS prevalence rates, large numbers of teachers, administrators and other educational employees are becoming infected, with substantial impacts on the supply and quality of education. An estimated 4–5 teachers die of AIDS each day in Zambia, for example, and an estimated 30 per cent of teachers in Malawi are infected with HIV (Commonwealth Secretariat, 2001). In 1999 alone, an estimated 860,000 primary school children in sub-Saharan Africa lost their teachers to AIDS (UNICEF, 2002). In addition, the consequences for the planning, administration and management of education are expected to be profound, and strategies for the organisation of the sector will require substantial re-thinking. The epidemic is likely to result not only in losses of education personnel but also in significant reductions in government funding for education, as economies decline and the direct and indirect consequences of AIDS-related sickness and death create competing priorities for the available resources.

At the same time, HIV/AIDS is also causing a substantial decline in the demand for education. Numerically, there will be far fewer children needing to be educated than was originally expected (over 25 per cent less in some countries) because fewer are being born and fewer are surviving to school age. Fewer children of school age are enrolling as a result of poverty, being orphaned, or the stigma of having an infected parent or other close relative. Children, especially girls and orphans, are also dropping out of schools in increasing numbers to take care of sick family members, or to support their families.

Overall, the available evidence indicates that HIV/AIDS is making the gender-based disparities that already exist in the education sector worse. In most cases these disadvantage girls in their access to quality education and disadvantage women in their employment opportunities as educators and administrators. As a result, many countries are likely to fail to meet the internationally agreed targets for gender equality in education and education for all. It is important to recognise that schools do not always represent safe environments, particularly for girls. A number of aspects of the school organisation and environment need to be addressed to reduce risk.

On the plus side, schools can play a positive role in helping learners and teachers to cope with the issue of HIV/AIDS. They can influence social attitudes and cultural norms acquired by young people. Alongside the family, peers, religion and the media, education plays a profoundly important part in the socialisation process. Education has been described as a 'social vaccine' against the epidemic since "the more education, the less HIV" (Loewenson and Whiteside, 2001). Schools also need to produce an adequate supply of educated people with the skills and training needed to support themselves, their families and communities against a background where there are increasing human resource shortages due to the devastating impact of HIV/AIDS.

In addition, schools have important roles to play as focal points for the community. Teachers, parent-teacher associations and governing bodies often command a degree of respect and authority that can be used to advantage in mobilising community action. Local strategies need to be developed that draw on these resources and supplement them by collaborations with NGOs, including women's organisations, and the private sector to mobilise action. This action can be used not only to support the school but also to ensure that information reaches as many people as possible in the community and that initiatives are taken to eliminate gender-based discrimination and inequality and create community solidarity in combating HIV/AIDS and making its effects less severe.

Policy/Action/Intervention

- Improve the access of girls to formal schooling.

- Introduce AIDS education for school children and their parents.

- Ensure women and men have information about their own bodies and education about HIV/AIDS and other STIs.

- Facilitate access to condoms for young people.

- Ensure that a life skills programme is implemented for young people in schools.

- Expand the life skills programme to young people out-of-school.

- Ensure safe transport to and from school for female pupils and teachers and safe school environments that avoid the possibility of sexual abuse or assault by other pupils, school staff, or unauthorised visitors to the school precincts.

- Prevent sexual relationships between staff and pupils, whether resulting from abuse or exploitation or as a means of obtaining financial or academic reward.

- Ensure that the infected and the affected are not excluded from education.

- Consider fee subsidies/exemptions to enable orphans to attend school.

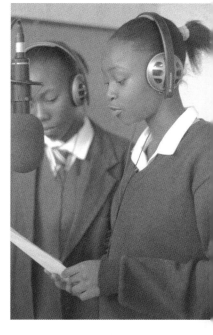

Two adolescent girls from a junior secondary school record their discussion on HIV/AIDS awareness and prevention in a booth at Radio Botswana.
UNICEF/HQ01-0173/Giacomo Pirozzi

Treatments for controlling HIV . . . remain inaccessible to most people living with HIV in developing countries.

> **Box 19: Responding to HIV/AIDS and Education (Vanuatu)**
>
> The Wan Smolbag Theatre in Vanuatu developed a play for primary schoolchildren – acted by a group of primary school dropouts – which explains how the body works, while a series of sketches addresses topics such as STIs. Plays for secondary schools have examined population growth, family planning and condom use; other theatre pieces have focused on teenage pregnancy, maternal health and HIV/AIDS. Wan Smolbag also publishes videos and papers with teachers' guides.
>
> *Source:* UNAIDS, 2001a

- Involve students in tertiary institutions in HIV/AIDS-related research and interventions.

Health

The epidemic has had a profound impact on health services in most of the affected countries. Bed occupancy has reached levels of 60–85 per cent. This has worsened the chronic shortage of equipment supplies and medicines, making it more difficult to provide basic health services. Illness and absenteeism of health staff has also had a major impact on health services. The ever-increasing cost of care through formal and traditional health systems can be overwhelming to the family. Despite the difficulties in the health care system, some useful responses, such as home care, that involve the participation of communities and the family, have been developed.

Treatments for controlling HIV, such as triple, double or combination antiretroviral therapy, have come into widespread use in the developed world over the past two years. Yet because of the cost (£10,000 per year) and difficulty in administering them, they remain inaccessible to most people living with HIV in developing countries. Possible reduction in cost using combinations of anti-viral and anti-cancer agents may help to make it possible for more affected people to receive

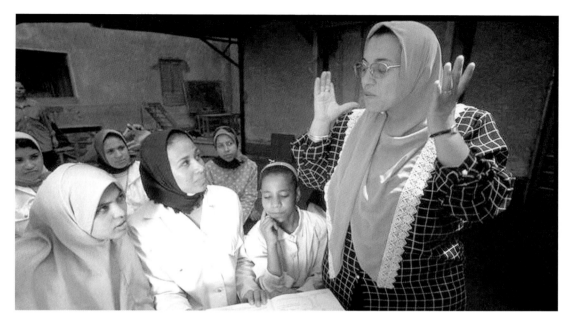

Health promotion at a women's group in Upper Egypt.
UNAIDS/G.Pirozzi

treatment. Studies of the benefits, and of possible ways in which these and other antiretroviral drugs can be made available in countries where the health budget is insufficient to meet basic health needs, are still being evaluated. Recent studies have also shown that a single dose of the antiretroviral, Nevirapine, given to an infected woman in labour, and another dose given to her baby within three days of birth, reduces the HIV transmission rate by half. This would potentially prevent some 300,000 to 400,000 babies per year being born infected with HIV. There are, however, ethical issues involved in providing a pregnant woman with treatment only to prevent transmission rather than for her own infection.

In places where sufficient resources cannot be mobilised for these costly drugs, people living with HIV/AIDS must have access to basic pain relief and treatment for 'simpler' opportunistic infections such as pneumonia and tuberculosis (UNDPI and UNAIDS, 2001). At the same time, it should be noted that although governments may argue that they cannot afford to increase their health budgets, this is often a matter of priorities. For example, the UN Independent Expert on Human Rights and Extreme Poverty, who has analysed the effects of poverty on the human rights of women, has pointed out that taking all developing countries together, military expenditure equals the combined total spending on health and education (Chinkin, 2001). Similarly, it has been argued that "about one eighth of the military budget in most countries [in Africa] would be enough to provide free antiretroviral drugs to all citizens living with HIV and AIDS" (Tlou, 2001).

Care and support for people living with HIV/AIDS can help to protect the health of the rest of the population by making prevention more effective. The majority of people do not know their HIV status, and the availability of care and treatment is likely to make more people seek voluntary testing and counselling. The Accelerating Access Initiative, launched by UNAIDS in May 2000, assists countries in implementing comprehensive packages of care. It aims both to make quality drugs more affordable and to collaborate with countries as they boost their capacity to deliver care, treatment and support. So far, 36 countries have taken advantage of this initiative (UNDPI and UNAIDS, 2001).

Box 20: Responding to HIV/ AIDS and Health (Zambia)

When the University Teaching Hospital in Zambia used to test children suspected of being HIV positive, they gave the test results only to mothers. Fathers who later learned that their children had HIV blamed the mothers and refused to be tested themselves. Now, when children show clinical symptoms suggesting HIV infection, the parents are called in together for counselling and both parents and the child are tested simultaneously. The test results are given to the parents together during additional counselling. This process has reduced blaming and tension between spouses.

Source: KIT, SAfAIDS and WHO, 1995

Policy/Action/Intervention

- Sensitise senior health planners, managers and service providers, to create a willing and supportive environment for the promotion of gender equality in the health sector.

- Integrate HIV/AIDS into all health promotion activities and services.

- Take action to ensure that women and girls, men and boys, have adequate access to sexual and reproductive health services.

- Ensure that both women and men have equal access to drugs for treating HIV/AIDS and opportunistic infections and to care.

- Keep the blood supply safe.

- Develop innovative methods of providing care to those infected and affected.

- Ensure that testing strategies address gender inequalities and possible stigmatisation, for example, counselling and testing couples before the woman gets pregnant.

Labour

HIV/AIDS brings about reduced labour quality and supply, more frequent and longer periods of absenteeism, and losses in skills and experience that result in a younger, less experienced workforce and subsequent production losses. These impacts intensify existing skills shortages and make training and benefits more costly (Loewensen and Whiteside, 2001). Along with lower productivity and profitability, tax contributions also decline while the need for public services increases (UNDPI and UNAIDS, 2001).

The rates of employment of women in the formal economy are generally lower than for men, since they are often engaged in subsistence farming as well as in their domestic and reproductive roles. However, recent data shows that women now comprise an increasing share of the world's labour force. In addition, the informal sector is a larger source of employment for women than for men and is growing.

Becoming HIV positive often has more economic impact on women than men. Women are more likely to lose employment in the formal sector and to suffer social ostracism and expulsion from their homes. On the other hand, self-employment can have positive advantages in resilience for women who become infected. When they are forced to become the main breadwinner due to their partner becoming infected, women who lack education and skills may be forced into

> **Box 21: Responding to HIV/AIDS and Labour (Tanzania)**
>
> In Tanzania, the national power company (TANESCO), local government authorities and health services have worked together to implement HIV prevention activities among migrant and local labourers working on the construction of a hydroelectric project at Kihansi Falls.
>
> *Source:* Commonwealth Secretariat, 2001

hazardous occupations, including sex work. These further increase their vulnerability.

The General Conference of the International Labour Organization (ILO), meeting in June 2001, recognised that HIV/AIDS had adversely impacted on economic growth and employment in all sectors of the economy. It adopted a Code of Practice on HIV/AIDS and the World of Work that provides practical guidelines to governments, employers and workers' organisations (as well as other stakeholders) for formulating and implementing appropriate workplace policy, prevention and care programmes, and for establishing strategies to address workers in the informal sector (ILO, 2001).

Policy/Action/Intervention

- Promote gender-responsive workplace prevention and care programmes in the private sector.

- Encourage companies to provide education on modes of transmission, prevention, factors driving the epidemic, the gender dimensions of HIV/AIDS and the implications of male sexual behaviour, and to promote STI treatment.

- Integrate HIV/AIDS prevention and control into companies' health policies.

- Develop workplace policies that are non-discriminatory.

- Encourage informal sector entrepreneurship and micro-credits, as well as community action groups and social welfare support mechanisms.

Law and justice

In many countries, women experience substantial discrimination in their legal status and treatment compared with men. This may include diminished rights to hold, inherit or dispose of property, to participate in democratic processes, or to make decisions about marriage or about the education of their children. HIV/AIDS is exacerbating the difficulties that women face and may make it difficult for them to exercise their rights to their property, employment, marital status and security. More women are now being widowed at a younger age and may be disinherited by the husband's relatives and unable to support themselves. They may also expect to die early themselves, yet be unable to provide for their children The legal environment can have a important impact on the quality of life for widows and orphans (Southern African AIDS Training Programme, 2001).

Sex work raises complex legal problems since, where this is illegal, sex workers are vulnerable to abuse and difficult to reach with STI/HIV prevention and support programmes (KIT/SAfAIDS/WHO, 1995). They may also resist seeking medical attention. Similarly, the stigma attached to homosexuality in many countries means that men who have sex with other men will avoid going to doctors and may feel forced to hide their sexual preference by getting married, thus putting their wives at risk.

Laws that can actively promote a supportive environment include those that protect the right to privacy; provide redress in the event of discrimination in employment, housing, access to health care, etc.; bar discrimination against people with HIV or their family or friends; protect the confidentiality of a person's HIV status; and require a person's consent to be given before HIV testing is undertaken (Hamblin, 1992). Legal protection has to be available in practice as well as in theory (i.e., widely publicised, accessible, etc.).

Policy/Action/Intervention

- Review the legal status of women to ensure that they have full and equal rights compared with men and that the protection of the law extends to those who become infected, orphaned or widowed as a result of HIV/AIDS.

In many countries, women experience substantial discrimination in their legal status and treatment compared with men.

- Review laws to ensure they support, rather than hinder, HIV/AIDS prevention efforts. This includes laws and policies affecting confidentiality, sex education, sex work, injecting drug use and homosexual behaviour.

- Formulate legal frameworks with the aim of eliminating all forms of violence against women and girls, including harmful traditional and cultural practices, abuse and rape, sexual harassment, battering and trafficking.

- Conduct sensitisation seminars and workshops for the legal profession and law enforcement officers to ensure that the legal provisions for equality are fully implemented.

- Incorporate HIV/AIDS awareness into legal training.

- Enact new laws as necessary that deal with specific problems raised by HIV/AIDS, such as: legal sanctions against persons knowingly infecting others; rights to confidentiality; and protection of employment, sickness benefits, pension rights and life insurance policies.

- Review laws relating to the status of commercial sex workers and homosexuals.

- Train police services to deal with sexual violence and abuse.

> ### Box 22: Responding to AIDS and the Law (India and South Africa)
>
> In India, the Lawyers Collective provides legal aid to those affected with HIV/AIDS and advocates for changes in the law to protect the human rights of people living with HIV/AIDS (PLHA) and to address stigma and discrimination. In South Africa, the AIDS Law Project and Lawyers for Human Rights produced a resource manual on HIV/AIDS and the law which has helped counsellors, lawyers, health workers, activists, unions and PLHA to address legal problems related to HIV/AIDS in a non-discriminatory way and to advocate for policies to protect the human rights of PLHA.
>
> *Source:* Commonwealth Secretariat, 2001

4. Case Studies of Gender-based Responses to Combating HIV/AIDS

Introduction

Programmes that promote HIV prevention by addressing gender equality, as well as the social and economic factors that put people at increased risk for infection, are more likely to succeed in changing behaviour, as can be seen from the case studies described below. The AIDS Vancouver and the Positive Women's Network (Canada), for example, provides an alternative research perspective which questioned the traditional focus on women's behaviours, such as sex workers' use of condoms or women's risk-taking behaviours in drug use. Instead, it addressed the reality of marginalised, excluded or 'forgotten' high-risk populations. Gender and culture were both addressed as determinants of health.

Gender-based research such as this, and other examples listed on the Canadian Women's Health Network website (see Chapter 5), demonstrate clearly the importance of listening to women's voices and addressing their lived realities in informing HIV/AIDS prevention campaigns. Applied HIV/AIDS research, conducted locally by researchers in co-operation with local communities, has considerable potential to influence national policy and promote action on the social factors that affect women's and men's health and wellbeing over their lifespan. This increases the likelihood of being able to target strategic interventions to high-risk populations, including sex workers.

One of the case studies focuses on this area – female prostitutes and HIV prevention programmes in Canada. Other studies address a number of different issues. From Africa comes a case study on marketing the female condom in Zimbabwe. This suggests that female condoms are providing new and additional protection from STIs/HIV to some study participants, though more research is needed. A case study of HIV counselling and testing among pregnant women in Canada offers best practices in this area, while involving men in preventing gender violence and HIV transmission is the focus of an international case study of a programme called Stepping Stones. This uses peer groups to help people translate information about prevention into behavioural change. Another innovative programme, called the School Without Walls, comes from Southern Africa and involves the transfer of local knowledge for HIV programming. The need to mobilise the community for effective control and prevention is also emphasised by a case study on sexual and reproductive health integration in Bangladesh. The final case study, from Canada, looks at gender differences in sexual health promotion among adolescents.

These case studies illustrate how a gender-based perspective on HIV/AIDS research, policy and programme will:

- respect women's and men's different perspectives and experiences;

- weave together research, policy and action in a meaningful way;

- hear the voices of women and men not typically heard in health research or health systems;

- explore strategies that build on the needs identified by HIV-positive men and women;

- address factors that influence the respective values and behaviours of women and men, particularly those residing in low income, economically marginalised, high-risk and hard to reach populations; and

- influence national public opinion through research and action that is targeted to specific policy audiences at the local, state/provincial and/or federal jurisdictions.

Case Study: Participatory Research with Marginalised Communities (Canada)

This project has played a big part in lifting my self-esteem, in getting me out there and getting a job and accepting a position in the help-

ing field … It's boosted my confidence and made me feel comfortable expressing how I really feel.

Research participant

Women's individual behaviour is often cited as the cause for their HIV infection or illness progression, for example, sex workers' use of condoms or risk-taking behaviour in drug use. HIV prevention strategies often target behaviour without exploring the larger factors that shape and inform it. In 1998, AIDS Vancouver and the Positive Women's Network initiated a research project that looked at women's risks from HIV infection and illness progression, using two main principles as a guide:

- Social and political factors form barriers to women's health, and should be explicitly explored along with potential strategies to overcome these barriers.

- The community's norms of whose voice gets heard and who is the 'expert' should be challenged.

Social and political factors form barriers to women's health, and should be explicitly explored along with potential strategies to overcome these barriers

Research focusing on behaviours assumes that individuals have enough power in their society to be able to change their behaviour and that they have choices. While this may be true for some individuals in some groups, social conditions reduce the options to a very narrow range for many people in marginalised groups. This is reflected in HIV statistics. It is the people at the bottom of the social and political hierarchy in their society who are most at risk from HIV/AIDS. For a woman living on welfare in a dangerous area, using valium or heroin or alcohol to cope, her risks are determined not by the right personal selection of a healthy option but instead by a socially-determined lack of options.

There are numerous social and political barriers that prevent women from taking care of their health. This fact was clearly understood and articulated by participants in the research. In looking at social barriers to health, the project hoped to re-orient the focus of research, examining the socio-

It is the people at the bottom of the social and political hierarchy in their society who are most at risk from HIV/AIDS.

economic conditions rather than women's behaviours and targeting social change in order to lessen the barriers to women's health.

The community's norms of whose voice gets heard and who is the 'expert' should be challenged

Several AIDS studies and consultations in Vancouver in recent years asked service providers about the risks and solutions for marginalised communities and asked members of marginalised communities only about their behaviours or lifestyle, not their ideas or suggestions for change. Many researchers used community members for their research, then took the information out for their own interpretation and profit but did not leave information or skills behind for the community. The project wanted to work with groups who had been researched a great deal but who had not been involved in creating knowledge in a meaningful way.

By sharing with women the tools and the means to do research, it was hoped that marginalised communities would have an opportunity to explore their definitions of the problems and their solutions, and use the information to take the kind of action they wanted to see happen. It was also hoped that their research and advocacy efforts might influence health policy and collaborative work with sympathetic policy-makers and health workers. If women from marginalised communities could use their research results as a tool to access decision-making bodies, perhaps they could then find allies in these decision-making bodies that would result in shared power and social change.

Phase One

The purpose of Phase One was problem identification. It used focus groups to gather information and, more importantly, to generate community interest and support. The project co-ordinator collaborated with other agencies to work with six different groups of women: Spanish-speaking immigrants and refugees; women with serious mental illness; First Nations and aboriginal women; HIV-positive women; current and former substance users; and lesbian/bisexual women. Each group looked at how specific social factors impact on their risk for HIV infection and illness progression, including:

- income;

- power in intimate relationships (meaning friends, partners, family);

- relationship with health care providers and health institutions.

Income

The study, like many others, found significant barriers to personal health and safety due to poverty. However, women talked not just about the lack of access to food and housing but also about the discrimination they experienced because of their poverty as a barrier to their health. The prevailing attitude that the poor must have done something wrong and deserve to suffer intensifies for many of them the guilt they already feel, so they do not ask for services that are rightfully theirs. This class discrimination erects additional barriers for those already living in poverty and further limits their health options.

Policy-makers must begin to see and understand that the standard of living maintained by welfare levels in Canada creates health risks not only due to material deprivations but also due to the shame of being poor in a wealthy land. Constructing affordable housing and providing extra money for good quality food are two examples of material benefits, but equally important is the shift required in how the 'non-poor' view those living in poverty.

Power in intimate relationships

Like numerous other studies, the research found that past and current experiences of abuse were linked to increased risk of HIV infection. Women also linked their experiences of abuse to ongoing poor health and shortened life spans. For example, an AIDS-defining illness might not be the most significant health risk for an HIV-positive woman in these communities. Instead, it might be a violent partner who assaults her; a long-standing drug addiction as a means to cope with memories of childhood abuse; or an inability to leave her home to seek medical treatment for weeks or months after a rape. Health

The study . . . found significant barriers to personal health and safety due to poverty.

Some women were taking their free prescription medications and selling them on the street in order to earn enough money to buy herbal or other alternative medicines.

risks of this type can form a web of barriers that makes it unlikely the woman would live long enough to develop an AIDS-defining illness.

Despite the innovative work done by some groups in Canada to document and take action on these issues, there is still need to raise the public's awareness. Policy-makers and public health educators have a potentially important role to play in helping to investigate and publicise the links between relationship abuse and HIV. Also, provision of adequate, long-term resources to women leaving abusive relationships (especially in rural areas) needs to be more actively linked to HIV prevention and support strategies.

Relationship with healthcare providers and health institutions

While there were stories of healthcare providers whose sincere caring had made a life-saving difference for women, there were also stories of appalling discrimination and the life-threatening consequences of inferior treatment. These point to the long-standing need to develop policy initiatives which will encourage ongoing training for health care providers regarding structures of power, privilege and oppression, in order to reduce discrimination against marginalised groups. Up-to-date HIV information also needs to be provided for non-specialist doctors so they are more comfortable with providing care and support to HIV-positive people.

Another barrier identified by women across all six focus groups was the lack of support from the mainstream medical establishment for access to alternative medicine and complementary therapies. HIV-positive women saw the pharmaceutical industry as controlling the treatment and research agenda of the 'AIDS establishment'. Some women were taking their free prescription medications and selling them on the street in order to earn enough money to buy herbal or other alternative medicines. Women and men will continue to use alternative and complementary therapies with or without their doctor's support or knowledge. It is therefore strongly suggested that the mainstream medical profession be encouraged to work with alternative and complementary healthcare professionals, integrating such research and information into their practice, and that the Canadian public healthcare system be amended to include the provision of alternative healthcare services and medicines.

Phase Two

After Phase One was completed, the project co-ordinator had established enough trust with women in the focus group communities to begin the second phase. This involved the training and support of peer researchers in order to further identify community needs and preferred strategies for change. A community-based educator was hired to work with the peer researchers using simple, accessible participatory methods. These focused not only on research skills but also on fostering bonding, communication and sharing between peer researchers, contributing to their empowerment as a group. After receiving training in one-to-one interviews and focus group facilitation, peer researchers took the information from Phase One back to other women in their self-identified home communities. They asked women what changes they wanted to see happen in order to reduce barriers to their health, as identified in the previous phase.

Through this process, combined with ongoing support and skills building, women gained a sense of ownership of the research. The project became theirs, not just the property of AIDS Vancouver and the Positive Women's Network. This was the first step in the transition from *community-based* research to *community-owned* research, and the stage at which staff began to learn more deeply about the meaning of changing the balance of power.

Recommendations

Sharing power must be encouraged at multiple levels of a project, whether research, prevention campaigns or whatever the level of involvement is with the community. The following suggestions seek to encourage power-sharing with communities, and can be implemented at local and national levels.

Networking: It is important to utilise links with other community agencies in order to share information and resources, share the work-load and involve the greatest possible number of community members. In this way, the project and its results do not become the 'property' of one agency. This can be a challenge when agencies have different agendas and perhaps also compete for funding. However, by involving other agencies in meaningful ways, sharing of power is role-modelled at the community agency level. Including a mix of people (for example from the community, local government, health professions, agency staff) will also challenge different pieces of the project, ensuring mutual education and increased potential for project integrity.

Involving members of the community: If a community is to increase its voice and power, then people must have a place in decision-making. However, the trap of 'tokenism' can arise due to differing levels of power. In Phase One, the project had only two seats reserved for community members on the advisory board; the other six were agency staff and health professionals. This had the effect of making the two HIV-positive women sometimes feel intimidated and silenced. There must be awareness of and sensitivity to these power dynamics, as well as a commitment to seek and develop innovative methods to solicit community involvement beyond the usual advisory boards and 'special committees'.

Working within the community: In order to facilitate the above, outreach services and sharing of resources are both important. Service providers need to get out of their offices and take their services to where women spend their time – the community centre, the church, the street – rather than expecting women to be able to come to their agencies. Outreach workers are crucial to a programme's link with a community, facilitating the community's communication of its needs. Communities also need resources in order to facilitate the communication of their needs and vision. Peer education and skills training, combined with encouragement to develop strong political analysis, give marginalised groups the tools to participate fully in the processes of learning about their needs and opportunities, and then take the action required to address them.

Changing the balance of power: Increased awareness and education can be shared among all members of the community.

This is the very essence of changing the balance of power. Working toward community empowerment, and challenging political and social systems, means changing the very nature of the current system. Hence, it can be helpful to remember to:

- *Invest in the long-term:* In-depth work with a community takes time and commitment. Prepare for this from the outset, putting in the supports and resources necessary to sustain staff and community members. If work is done too quickly (for example to meet a funder's short-term project goal), this can leave the community in worse shape than before the project started.

- *Prepare for conflict:* Conflict will naturally arise when different groups are brought together. Skilled facilitation is required to work through conflict, not around it.

- *Ask whose needs are being met:* The agency's priority may not be the community's priority. When community members are asked to define their priorities, they may want to act on needs other than those identified by funders, agencies or academic institutions. Empowerment means letting the marginalised communities take the lead and giving them the skills and resources to do so.

Conclusion

Truly representative community consultation and mobilisation is a slow and complex process. It is important to take the time to develop community voices and listen for what is being said (not just what the researchers want to hear). Because of this, the sense of ownership and empowerment felt by all members of the team, and the depth and diversity of the information gathered, has created a very rich research project. It is hoped that by targeting barriers in social and political systems and supporting community empowerment, the project is contributing to a process of change that will continue long after the research is finished, and will sustain real change in the health and dignity of marginalised communities.

Source: Tolson and Kellington, 2001

Truly representative community consultation and mobilisation is a slow and complex process.

Case Study: HIV Prevention Programmes and Female Prostitutes (Canada)

Introduction

During the earliest days of the HIV epidemic, female prostitutes were seen as 'vectors of transmission'. Many believed that prostitutes would be the mechanism through which HIV would spread from the gay community to the heterosexual community. There were calls to quarantine female sex workers, or to license prostitutes and to have the license tied to being free of sexually transmitted infections (STIs) including HIV. At the same time, there was also opposition to such demands, particularly from the gay community and prostitutes' rights organisations who strongly disagreed with the portrayal of female prostitutes as the problem.[1]

The almost exclusive focus on female prostitutes as the 'cause' of the spread of HIV represented a fundamentally flawed assumption about the nature of the relationship between female prostitute and client within the North American context. Indeed, the assumption that multiple high-risk sexual services were being provided without the use of condoms was not borne out by research. As research in the past 15 years has consistently indicated, most female prostitutes within North America (as well as parts of Europe and Australia) typically use condoms with clients, and rates of HIV are relatively low among non-injection drug using prostitutes (Hancock, 1998; Jackson et al., 1992; Seidlin et al., 1988). In fact, most North American prostitutes are now characterised as 'safer sex professionals' because of their role in ensuring the use of condoms when providing a sexual service.

Incorrect assumptions about the nature of the female prostitute-client relationship continue to exist, however. Many HIV-related policies and programmes are based on the notion that the female prostitute is, and should be, the one responsible for safer sex. The prostitute is viewed as selling a commodity – sexual services – which are purchased 'freely' on the market, and because she is selling the service she is respon-

---

[1] 'Prostitutes' here refers specifically to women who exchange sex for money or in kind and does not include women in the sex trade industry who exclusively provide other services such as phone talk sex.

sible for the health and safety of the client (Davidson, 1998; Jackson and Hood, in press). As such, most HIV prevention efforts target female prostitutes with HIV education, providing access to condoms and often other medical services. However, this focus fails to take a critical look at the nature of the sex trade industry, the relations that maintain the industry and women's dependence on the sale of sexual services. It also ignores the class, race and gender inequities that play a fundamental role in women's entrance into prostitution and their vulnerability to HIV.

Within much of North America there is a double standard in terms of female prostitution . . .

Female prostitution and the double standard

Within much of North America there is a double standard in terms of female prostitution or women who work in the sex trade industry. On the one hand, there is a dominant moral disdain for the selling of one's body to multiple customers. This disdain is represented in the criminalisation of activities related to the woman's role in prostitution (Davidson, 1998). Women who engage in the sale of sexual services are arrested for soliciting and constantly have to guard against police arrest, especially if they are street prostitutes – the most visible form of prostitution. On the other hand, the clients (or 'Johns') of female prostitutes typically do not undergo constant police scrutiny. Although in some centres there are instances where clients have been arrested and sentenced to 'John' school that is intended to deter them from frequenting prostitutes, it is typically the woman prostitute who is stigmatised and punished, not her male clients. This means that more often than not it is the woman who suffers the economic consequences related to arrest, thus contributing to the economic hardships that have led many women into prostitution in the first place.

Female prostitutes are also often blamed for the violence perpetuated by clients, and frequently there is a weak, if any, response by the police and other authorities to such violence. At the same time, there is state support for some prostitution-related activities (which are often male-owned and operated), such as escort services and body-rub parlours. Typically, these businesses are provided with licenses to operate, and those

A double standard also underlines many HIV prevention programmes and policies in Canada.

involved in such activities profit from the women's work of selling sexual services, yet it is the women who take the greatest risks in terms of violence perpetuated by clients (Alexander, 1998; Jackson and Hood, in press). Some women who work as street prostitutes are forced – either overtly or covertly – to provide much of their earnings to 'pimps', while many women who work as 'escorts' are also required to provide a large percentage of their earnings to the owners of these establishments.

HIV-prevention programmes/policies and the double standard

A double standard also underlines many HIV prevention programmes and policies in Canada. Prevention programmes do not typically target male clients even though these men may be as 'sexually active' as female prostitutes, visiting multiple women for both paid and unpaid sexual services. This double standard is especially problematic given that research indicates that when condoms are not utilised during the prostitute-client relationship, it is frequently because of the clients' resistance to condom use. Such resistance can take many different forms, from subtle coercion to more overt forms of violence. Regardless of the form, however, this represents a risk of HIV for female prostitutes.

Women also report being raped by clients, which once again points to the serious inequities between prostitute and client. It is also a situation that makes it impossible for the women to be 'safer sex professionals'. Many within the legal profession, as well as much of the public, believe that female prostitutes who are raped are 'asking for it' because of their work. This reveals a serious misunderstanding concerning rape, which is forced sexual relations against one's will and takes place because of gross power inequities in gender relations. Given this lack of understanding, and the stigma that many female prostitutes face when they attempt to report a rape, many rapes of female prostitutes are unreported and many women endure this violence and the long-term consequences of the violence without needed supports and services.

Clients also utilise economic incentives in an attempt to

ensure sexual services without the use of condoms – incentives that some women find difficult to resist because of their desperate economic need. In some instances this need is related to an alcohol or drug addiction, found to be quite prevalent among female prostitutes. Tremendous barriers confront women with addictions seeking treatment. These include the waiting times for accessing programmes, the lack of economic and social support for children when the women are in treatment, and the poor attitudes of some counsellors who are not sensitive to the women's situation and their work as prostitutes. The prevailing attitude is that drug use is a legal issue rather than a medical problem and this has been a major stumbling block to the establishment of needed treatments and treatment centres, as well as to many women seeking treatment. Many pregnant women and women with children are afraid to admit drug use and to seek help owing to the 'well-founded belief' that they will lose their babies (Whynot, 1998).

Just as women have traditionally been responsible for birth control and the unintended pregnancies resulting from birth control failures, female prostitutes are typically viewed as responsible for keeping the trade safe from STIs, including HIV. In many instances women take on this role because of the importance of maintaining their own health and wellbeing (not only so that they remain healthy but also so that they can continue to care for and financially support their families). However, there are contexts when condoms are not used, as noted above, and at times condoms break. In such instances the women, not the clients, are typically blamed and stigmatised for the consequences. Furthermore, although it is widely believed that HIV-infected female prostitutes should not be working, calls to have HIV-infected men who frequent prostitutes barred from doing so are not heard.

. . . although it is widely believed that HIV-infected female prostitutes should not be working, calls to have HIV-infected men who frequent prostitutes barred from doing so are not heard.

HIV prevention programmes/policies and the private sphere

To date, in Canada, most HIV prevention programmes have focused almost exclusively on ensuring condom use within prostitutes' working lives with male clients. Relatively little attention has been given to women's private lives and their

Most HIV-prevention programmes are not organised to address the general health and wellbeing of female prostitutes.

risks of HIV infection within this sphere of their lives when having sexual relations with men. However, many have noted that female prostitutes' greatest risk may be when having sexual relations with private partners (for example, a spouse or a boyfriend) who is an injection drug user because of the fact that typically condoms are not used outside of the work setting.

For many prostitutes condoms are associated with work and there is often a resistance to using them when having sexual relations with someone other than a client. Some women have noted that a condom interferes with the closeness of a private relationship exactly because of the use of condoms with clients. Condoms with clients represent both a physical and psychological barrier and this means that there is little interest in using them when one wants to be emotionally close to one's partner.

At the same time, when prostitutes do feel they would like to use condoms with a boyfriend or spouse because they believe that they are at high risk of HIV or other STIs, they are sometimes fearful of even broaching the topic for fear of negative repercussions. Some women have reported that their male partner would be terribly offended if the issue of condom use was raised because it would represent the client-prostitute relationship rather than an intimate relationship. This points to the fact that safer sex is not safe if it has the potential to challenge a relationship with a significant partner who might become violent.

Conclusion

Since the 1980s, many HIV-focused policies and programmes have been developed that were aimed at prostitutes. Numerous and varied educational programmes now exist in many centres, and prostitutes are frequently provided with free condoms, access to counselling services and so forth. However, such efforts are fundamentally aimed at ensuring that prostitutes remain free from HIV (as well as other STIs), in order to ensure that clients are safe from STIs and can pursue their leisure experiences without fear of HIV. Most HIV-prevention programmes are not organised to address the general health and wellbeing of female prostitutes. The women are viewed primarily as 'workers' rather than as women who enter the sex trade industry often because of economic need that is a product of systemic inequalities based on class, gender and race. For a large number of women who work in the sex trade industry, their vulnerability to HIV is rooted in the fact that they are economically disadvantaged and their poverty is directly related to gender, racial, ethnic and other inequalities.

Many women enter the sex trade industry because of poor employment opportunities and lack of work skills. In many instances, women who work in prostitution have experienced a history of child abuse – physical, sexual and/or emotional – that has led them to leave home at an early age. They thus lost the chance to complete their education with family support. Attempts to continue their education are extremely difficult and more often than not thwarted because of the economic costs of education and maintaining themselves financially. A number of women living on social assistance are unable to provide for themselves and/or their children. This makes the sex trade industry an attractive option both because it allows them to augment their income and because it provides work opportunities in a situation where they do not possess the education and skills to otherwise obtain a decent wage.

Clearly, programmes and policies are needed to tackle the underlying issues that are often precursors to women entering the sex trade industry and that keep them tied to this work even when it is dangerous and risky to their health. The socio-economic conditions that make women vulnerable to HIV – lack of power within male-female relationships, economic dependency, drug and alcohol addictions – need to be addressed. Women require access to educational and work opportunities and affordable housing and childcare. Policies are needed to ensure economic security for women and their children, as well as access to non-judgmental counselling and legal and medical services, regardless of their work. Women who find themselves working in the sex trade industry require the same level of protection as other women, and should not have to endure emotional abuse from professionals by being labelled as 'deviant', 'immoral', or 'unfit mothers'. These labels and the stigma associated with them only work to make women feel inferior, and fearful of obtaining needed services that might reduce their vulnerability to HIV.

For a large number of women who work in the sex trade industry, their vulnerability to HIV is rooted in the fact that they are economically disadvantaged and their poverty is directly related to gender, racial, ethnic and other inequalities.

It is also important that women who work or have worked in the sex trade industry take part in the development of policies and programmes to address the inequities women face. Providing them with a voice in the planning of programmes and development of policies will help to ensure the implementation of social changes that will directly benefit these women. It will also help to empower the women, most of whom have lived much of their lives outside the realm of programme development and policy decision-making.

Source: Jackson, 2001

Case Study: Marketing the Female Condom (Zimbabwe)

The female condom is a relatively new product that prevents pregnancy and sexually transmitted infections (STIs). The World Health Organization (WHO) estimates a 5 per cent annual accidental pregnancy rate associated with perfect use of the female condom, compared to 3 per cent with the male condom. A study on contraceptive efficacy suggests that perfect use of the female condom also reduces the annual risk of becoming infected with HIV by more than 90 per cent among women who have intercourse twice weekly with an infected male. This is similar to the level of protection offered by the male condom.

The female condom may also prove to be an HIV protection option over which women have more control. Many women may be unable or unwilling to negotiate male condom use with their sexual partners because of prevailing gender-related inequalities, norms and roles that exist in many societies.

In 1996, based on the positive findings of acceptability trials and as a result of advocacy efforts by the Women and AIDS Support Network, the Zimbabwe National AIDS Co-ordination Programme (NACP) of the Ministry of Health and Child Welfare invited Population Services International (PSI) to initiate a five-year female condom social marketing programme in Zimbabwe. The programme was launched in 1997.

To avoid the stigma associated with STI/HIV prevention, the female condom is marketed as a family planning product, a 'contraceptive sheath' under the brand name Care™. The product's original marketing slogans included "The care contraceptive sheath is for caring couples" and "For women and men who care". The female condom was initially sold through selected pharmacies and clinics at a heavily subsidised retail price of US$0.24 for a box of two. Distribution has since expanded to other urban outlets, including large supermarkets and convenience stores.

Research

As experience with the female condom in Zimbabwe and other countries increases, a number of research questions has arisen about its use and its potential for STI/HIV reduction. Answers to these questions (for example, who uses the female condom, with whom and why?) have important implications for reproductive health programmes. Currently, the female condom is a relatively expensive product, priced at approximately ten times the cost of a male condom. From a programme and policy standpoint, the decision to introduce this product in a given country on a wide scale implies significant financial costs. The introduction of heavily subsidised and relatively inexpensive female condoms in Zimbabwe through a social marketing programme has provided large numbers of urban women with easy access to this product. So the situation in Zimbabwe allowed the Horizons Project and PSI to address critical research questions with a fairly large number of respondents about female condom use under real life conditions.

The study used a combination of quantitative and qualitative methods. An intercept survey was conducted with women and men exiting urban sales outlets that carry both Protector Plus™ male condoms and Care™ female condoms. In total, 493 female condom users, 633 male condom users and 624 non-users were included in the study. Male and female users of the female condom also participated in in-depth interviews and focus groups.

Results

Who uses the female condom?
Users are generally in their mid- to late-twenties and, compared to male condom users and non-users of either method,

have higher levels of education and access to household resources. Among women, more users of the female condom are unmarried and are primary breadwinners in their households compared to users of male condoms and non-users. The vast majority of men and women had used the male condom at least once before trying the female condom. More than half of male users, but only 17 per cent of female users, reported having more than one sexual partner within the last year. Use of the female condom is higher within the context of marriage or regular partnerships rather than casual or commercial partnerships.

Reasons for female condom use
Novelty or experimentation and pregnancy prevention were primary reasons for the initial use of the female condom. However, a third of men and 21 per cent of women reported STI/HIV prevention as a motivator for trying it.

Perceptions of, and problems with, the female condom
Users perceived the female condom to be effective and reliable both as an STI/HIV prevention method and a contraceptive method. But 30 per cent of men and 57 per cent of women reported some difficulty with use, such as problems with insertion, discomfort during sex and excess lubrication.

Negotiation of the female condom
Both male and female users concurred that women, more than men, initiate dialogue about using the female condom, decide on its use and procure the product. However, a considerable percentage of both male and female users reported that both partners jointly decided to use it. Focus group and in-depth interview data revealed that while some women, particularly married women, were interested in using the female condom for disease prevention, they were not comfortable discussing this openly with their partner. Some 13 per cent of women reported using the female condom without their partners' knowledge. While this suggests that for some women the female condom can be totally under their control, in the vast majority of cases it requires communication with and cooperation from a woman's partner.

Nearly a fourth of women and 15 per cent of men said that one of their partners opposed female condom use. While most said they used a male condom instead, about half the married women whose partner opposed using the female condom had unprotected sex.

Consistency of female condom use

Overall, about 15 per cent of women and men reported always using the female condom. Consistent use was reported much less frequently with spouses than with regular partners outside marriage. Among those who had used both the female and male condom, approximately 80 per cent of men said they intended to use both methods in future. A greater proportion of women said they would use the female condom again (68 per cent) rather than the male condom (54 per cent). Married women were less likely than single women to report continued use of either barrier method.

Increased STI/HIV protection among some female condom users

Twenty-seven per cent of married women had never used a male condom before they used the female condom, and 20 per cent of consistent female condom users reported that they were not consistent male condom users before trying the female condom.

Continued male condom use among female condom users

Of inconsistent female condom users who have used the male condom, 93.8 per cent reported continued use of the male condom. Female condom users often alternated the use of male and female condoms. Women reported using female condoms when their husbands came home late at night or when they suspected infidelity. Also, some men reported using female condoms with their wives and regular partners while continuing to use male condoms with casual partners and sex workers.

Policy implications

The female condom has been used within marriage or a regular partnership and among consistent users, primarily as a family planning method which reflects the aims of the social marketing campaign. Single women and married men with outside

An important issue for programme planners is ensuring access to the female condom for people from all economic and educational strata.

partners seem to benefit most from its introduction. These are important groups to reach in a country such as Zimbabwe, which has a high prevalence of HIV in the general population.

An important issue for programme planners is ensuring access to the female condom for people from all economic and educational strata. If significantly greater percentages of people with higher socio-economic status or more formal education continue to use the product at higher rates, then the price of the condom may be too high. It is also possible that special support services may be needed to facilitate access, negotiation or correct use of the female condom among people with lower levels of resources and education.

Married women have particular needs that have to be addressed in future campaigns and educational programmes. Many married women perceive themselves to be at risk of HIV infection but do not use any barrier method. Among female condom users, married women are more likely than single women to encounter partner resistance to the female condom and less likely to report future use.

Face-to-face contact – with partners, friends, relatives or health professionals – was found to be important for motivating female condom use. Training both peer educators as well as clinicians and pharmacists to provide women and men with information and support services about the product may be an effective means of increasing correct and continued use. Also, female condom programming must assist users, in particular women, to be prepared for negotiation and agreement of use with partners. They must be equipped with the necessary skills and tools.

Data from this study suggests that female condoms are providing new and additional protection from STIs/HIV to some study participants. More research is needed to more accurately assess the female condom's contribution to increasing the incidence of protected sex among women and men in Zimbabwe.

Source: Kerrigan et al., 2000

Case Study: HIV Counselling and Testing among Pregnant Women: Best Practices (Canada)

Introduction

In Canada, women of childbearing age (15–44 years) accounted for approximately 79 per cent of the total AIDS cases among adult women reported to the Laboratory Centre for Disease Control, Health Canada, to the end of 1999 (Health Canada, 2000d). Of the 196 paediatric AIDS cases reported by that date, the majority (78 per cent) were attributed to parent-to-child transmission (PTCT) (Health Canada, 2000e). PTCT can occur in the mother's uterus prior to birth, during birth at the time of labour and delivery, and following birth through breastfeeding. Other factors that can increase the risk of transmission include maternal viral load, mode of delivery, timing of delivery after rupture of membranes and length of time breastfeeding.

Despite these facts, offering voluntary counselling and testing (VCT)[2] to pregnant women for HIV was not a public health policy objective to prevent the perinatal spread of HIV prior to 1994. Before this, HIV testing among pregnant women was provided either at the request of the pregnant women or on the judgement of their doctors. However, the results were then published of a randomised clinical trial of antiretroviral medication provided to mothers during the second or third trimester, during labour and delivery, and to their newborns for six weeks. These showed a two-thirds reduction in PTCT and caused the role of HIV testing in pregnancy to be rethought. (Connor E.M., Sperling R.S., Gelber R. et al., 1994). Further Canadian studies have shown antiretroviral therapy to be effective in reducing PTCT rates even lower than the eight per cent achieved in the trial (Forbes, J., Burdge, D.R., Money, D., 1997; Lapointe, 1998).

Although increased attention has been focused on the issue of the prevention of PTCT, most studies in the area have been quantitative in nature (i.e., they have been mainly concerned with looking at the numbers of pregnant women undergoing HIV testing). Little work has been done to investigate pregnant women's experiences with antenatal HIV testing from a qualitative perspective.

The present study was formulated to explain some of the gaps in our current knowledge regarding HIV VCT among pregnant women in Canada. More specifically, it aimed to pro-

Parent-to-child transmission [of HIV] can occur in the mother's uterus prior to birth, during birth at the time of labour and delivery, and following birth through breastfeeding.

---

[2]While this article uses the UNAIDS terminology of VCT, it is clear that HIV counselling and testing of women in this study was not always perceived as voluntary.

vide timely information from pregnant women to inform a federal position on an effective antenatal HIV counselling and testing policy for Canadian women. The goal was to document pregnant women's experiences of HIV testing in pregnancy and, based on these experiences, their perceptions of best practices regarding HIV counselling and testing.

Additionally, this national study allows for a comparison of the application and acceptability of current prenatal HIV testing policies in three provinces: Alberta, Ontario and Nova Scotia. In Canada, HIV testing programmes are the responsibility of provincial and territorial governments. There are no national recommendations or national policy guidelines in this area and, as a result, there are a range of different policies. The provinces were selected for this study because they had different approaches. In Alberta, the provincial policy offers an opt-out option, which essentially allows for all pregnant women to be routinely tested as part of the prenatal screening programme unless they specifically decline this. In Ontario, all pregnant women and women contemplating pregnancy are offered the opportunity for HIV counselling and testing. And in Nova Scotia, the provincial guidelines have recently changed from a policy suggesting HIV counselling and testing at the discretion of the physician to one suggesting that HIV counselling and testing should be offered to all pregnant women.

Methods

A total of 105 pregnant women, 35 from each province, was interviewed regarding their antenatal HIV counselling and testing experiences. The stratified sample of women in each case included Aboriginal women, women from HIV-endemic countries, visible minority women, women who would be considered to be at high risk for HIV infection, women considered to be at low risk and women who inject drugs. With the woman's consent, each interview was audio-taped and then transcribed and analysed to determine the types of issues women experience in relation to HIV counselling and testing during their pregnancy. The interview followed a guided conversational format, which allowed the pregnant women to elaborate on a number of key, interrelated issues. These included whether HIV testing had been offered, how it was offered and what were the women's assessments of best practices for HIV counselling and testing grounded in their own experiences.

Results

Preliminary findings show clear evidence that the established Canadian principles of voluntary HIV counselling and testing are not always maintained by programmes that offer to test women during pregnancy. While the majority of the women interviewed did accept testing when it was offered, many reported that they did not experience the offer to test as voluntary and did not feel that they had given their specific informed consent to be tested. Many women interviewed also reported that they had not been given adequate information to assess the risks and benefits of HIV and testing for themselves or for their unborn child.

In Alberta, where all pregnant women are routinely tested for HIV as part of the prenatal screening programme or other pregnancy-related tests (with the option to opt out), only 2.4 per cent of pregnant women declined testing during the second year of the programme. None of the women interviewed for this study had declined testing. However, many of the women either had no prior knowledge that they would be tested for HIV or were not informed about the test. If they were informed about the test, they were not presented with the option of declining. Nevertheless, all the women indicated that they were pleased that their doctor had included the HIV test among the prenatal tests that were ordered and would have agreed to the test if they had been given the option. They also added that they wanted to know about the testing even though it was routine. Furthermore, many of the women who participated in the study had had previous HIV testing and although they believed that they were still HIV negative they agreed to have the test since it was routine.

In Nova Scotia, where it is recommended that testing should be offered to all pregnant women, there were very few refusals of the test among study participants. This may reflect the fact that some women being testing for HIV either do not know it or do not feel comfortable asking their physician why the test is being offered to them. In addition, women who per-

. . . the established Canadian principles of voluntary HIV counselling and testing are not always maintained by programmes that offer to test women during pregnancy.

ceived themselves to be knowledgeable about HIV risk tended to decline testing when it was offered since they felt they knew their risks better than their physicians. Variability was found in the offer of testing by social class or ethnicity. For example, rural Aboriginal women were more likely to have been tested than were white women. Also, very few women interviewed in Nova Scotia felt that they had been given adequate pre- and post-test counselling or information regarding the use of the test results. Several women commented that they had wanted to do whatever their physician suggested regarding prenatal blood tests, believing that they were doing what was best for the baby. Some women also commented that they did not feel comfortable questioning or refusing the recommendations of their physicians to take the test for fear of possibly receiving sub-standard health care at subsequent appointments.

In Ontario, where all pregnant women and women contemplating pregnancy are offered the opportunity for HIV counselling and testing, some women have refused the offer of the test. Reasons for refusal centre on a previous history of accessing HIV testing outside pregnancy or their concerns regarding the use of the test results. Some women declined testing, as in Nova Scotia, based on their own assessment of their behavioural susceptibility to HIV infection, often confirmed by previous negative results; others declined simply because they were regularly tested either as blood donors or as part of their annual physical examination.

Discussion

Grounded in their own personal experiences, the women interviewed recommended developments in policy and practice which would ensure that prenatal programmes encompass HIV testing in a manner which is sensitive to both the needs of the pregnant woman as well as the prevention of HIV transmission. Several women remarked on how the focus for HIV testing during pregnancy is related to the foetus and not to the pregnant woman's wellbeing *per se*. In addition, it was felt by a number of women that removing the exceptional nature of HIV testing during pregnancy may help to reduce the stigma that is still often associated with HIV testing at other points across a woman's lifespan.

In terms of best practices, most of the women interviewed in Nova Scotia felt that their physicians were the individuals best suited to offer HIV testing in their pregnancies. However, they also pointed out the need for greater standardisation of pre- and post-test counselling to reduce the variability in the way the test is offered to pregnant women and under what circumstances. Some women interviewed felt that they either had sufficient levels of HIV knowledge prior to their physician suggesting the test or were given this in the course of their pre-natal care. Several others, however, felt that more emphasis ought to be placed on providing information on the treatment options for women who are found to be HIV positive during pregnancy. Very few women commented on having access to any information on antiretroviral treatment to reduce the risk of transmission to their baby, leading some women to report that they would abort the foetus rather than risk carrying it to term and potentially giving birth to an HIV infected baby.

There was consensus among those interviewed that preventing PTCT is an important issue and that additional information and resources could be used to increase the visibility of the purpose, the procedure and the use of the test results. In addition to the pamphlet produced by the Canadian Public Health Association on women and AIDS, it was felt that other pamphlets, videos, websites or toll-free hotlines are needed, particularly for those women who live in more remote areas of the province.

In Ontario, most pregnant women interviewed supported the provincial policy. They saw the offer of an HIV test in pregnancy as the first step in accessing, if necessary, the choice of treatment for themselves and preventive interventions to reduce transmission to their unborn children. However, many women were very clear that pregnancy was not the most appropriate time to raise the issue of HIV infection with women or to offer testing. Pre-conception – before deciding on pregnancy or at the time of an annual pap smear or physical examination, for example – was favoured by many women because knowledge of their HIV status would have been a factor in their decision to become pregnant. Other perspectives on the timing of the offer of antenatal HIV testing included the idea that the issue should be raised early enough in the pregnancy to allow the pregnant woman access to a range of options,

Very few women commented on having access to any information on antiretroviral treatment to reduce the risk of transmission to their baby . . .

. . . women wanted information about how women can contract HIV and how it is transmitted to the foetus.

which might include termination. It was also suggested that the discussion around the offer to test for HIV should be carried out over several visits, which would allow for personal reflection and discussion with the woman's family and partner as appropriate. An issue of particular importance for women in Ontario was the recommendation that HIV testing should be the focus of a prenatal visit and not combined with other routine tests offered in pregnancy, in particular the offer of maternal serum screening.

As in the two other provinces, their doctor was the first choice of most Ontario women to raise the issue of the opportunity to test for HIV in pregnancy. For some women, their doctor was their preferred health care professional as they felt that the discussion around HIV testing would remain confidential; for others it was because they had an established relationship with their doctor based on trust. However, some women would choose the health care provider who is most accessible to them in terms of the time they have available and suggested nurses attached to physicians' practices, public health nurses and midwives.

Finally, most of the women in Ontario, as in the other two provinces, wanted much more information than was offered to them before they took the test. In addition to describing the information they needed from their health care provider, they made suggestions for the contents of a brochure to be made available to every pregnant woman or woman considering pregnancy in Ontario. They suggested that this could be distributed at the point of sale of feminine hygiene products and pregnancy home-testing kits.

In Alberta too, women's responses provided further insights into best practices for HIV counselling and testing. A few women also identified nurses, in addition to physicians, as possible people to deliver HIV VCT. They felt that nurses have more time and would be more likely to be more accessible than physicians, particularly in more remote areas of the province. As well as information about treatment, women wanted information about how women can contract HIV and how it is transmitted to the foetus. Although Alberta has produced brochures with this information, most of the women in the study had not seen them. This was also the case with respect to the brochures produced in Ontario. The majority of the women in Alberta supported the routine testing programme and several advocated mandatory testing. They noted that the routine nature of the testing resulted in less stigma because it was less stressful and embarrassing than having to request the test. However, many women said they would ask for an HIV test if they had concerns.

In order for pregnant women to increase control over their own health and that of their unborn children, there is clear value in all pregnant women being afforded the opportunity to know their HIV status. However, in efforts to reduce PTCT, it is essential that a pregnant woman's needs and rights to best practices in HIV counselling and testing are protected. Failure to attend to the quality or variability of the experiences of HIV counselling and testing in pregnancy will result in programmes that fail to increase testing acceptance rates and fail to provide women with the resources they need to make the best decisions for themselves and for their children.

Source: Leonard, Gahagan, Doherty and Hankins, 2001

. . . violence against women is a leading cause of death globally, accounting for more deaths among females aged 15–44 than traffic accidents, malaria, cancer or war.

Case Study: Involving Men in Preventing Gender Violence and HIV Transmission (International)

Stepping Stones targets men, particularly young men, and works with them and women to redefine gender norms and encourage healthy sexuality.

Geeta Rao Gupta (Gupta, 2000a)

HIV/AIDS has reversed hard-earned development gains and introduced into society new fault lines for discrimination and violation of individual and community rights. At the same time, violence against women is a leading cause of death globally, accounting for more deaths among females aged 15–44 than traffic accidents, malaria, cancer or war. HIV and gender violence are linked. Rape and other forms of sexual violence carry transmission risks, and the threat of violence inhibits the ability to talk openly about sexual issues such as condom use.

Some of the biggest challenges to preventing gender violence and HIV transmission are:

- *Tackling silence, denial and stigma.* Shame and fear lead to unwillingness to address the issues openly.

- *Challenging the acceptability of gender inequality in sexual relationships and decision-making.* Too often, culture is used as an excuse to justify a whole range of practices and structures that violate women's human rights. Traditional social and cultural expectations harm men as well, by denying them the opportunity to develop skills of nurturing, caring, communication and non-violent conflict resolution.

- *Moving from awareness to behaviour change.* Many interventions and campaigns are built on the false assumption that information leads automatically to behaviour change. There is insufficient support to enable individuals and communities to bridge the gap between knowledge and practice.

To meet these challenges, Stepping Stones was first developed in 1995 in Uganda. It has since been used by over 2,000 organisations in 104 countries worldwide. Local groups have translated and adapted it for their own use in many different countries, including Sri Lanka (Sinhala), Cambodia (Khmer), Russia, urban South Africa, Tanzania (Ki-swahili), Argentina (Spanish) and Mozambique (Portuguese). It is based on the following principles:

- The best solutions are those developed by people themselves.

- Men and women each need private time and space with their peers to explore their own needs and concerns about relationships and sexual health.

- Behaviour change is much more likely to be effective and sustained if the whole community is involved.

Rather than concentrating on individuals or segregated 'risk' groups, Stepping Stones works through groups of peers of the same gender and similar age (older women, older men, younger women and younger men). The groups work separately much of the time so that they have a safe, supportive space for talking about intimate issues and then periodically meet together to share insights. All the work is based on people's own experiences, and the use of role-play, drawing, song and dance means that everyone can take part, without needing any formal education background.

The workshop sessions

It is suggested that a total of 18 separate workshop sessions be held over a period of 9–12 weeks in a community. Spreading the sessions over several weeks like this enables community members who want to join the workshop to put what they have learned into practice between sessions. The sessions cover four themes:

Co-operation and communication. This helps each peer group to bond together and creates a safe, friendly atmosphere in which to explore sensitive issues. The facilitator or trainer of each group is the same gender and age as the members so that everyone feels comfortable as peers.

Relationships, HIV and safer sex. The men's and women's groups each have a chance to assess their own priorities in sexual health and family life, in the context of greater understanding of their potential vulnerability to HIV. Domestic violence – often linked to alcohol abuse – is an issue frequently highlighted by both men's and women's groups.

What influences us to behave the way we do. This includes, crucially, society's expectations of men and women (gender roles) which are often closely linked to cultural tradition.

How to practice and sustain change. The final sessions of the training workshop address "ways in which we can change" and explore assertiveness skills and non-violent conflict resolution.

The culmination of the process is a 'special request' from each peer group to the whole community, presented in the form of a role play, which illustrates the change each group sees as a top priority. The issues raised are then discussed by everyone present. This enables young women, for example, to present the dilemmas which they face with 'sugar daddies' who pursue them for sexual favours in return for school fees; or for older men to present the loss of self-esteem that turns them to drinking when they are made redundant. This sharing between groups enable everyone in the community to develop more awareness of the needs and difficulties of others around them, as well as increasing their own self-esteem and self-respect through having their own needs appreciated more clearly. This reciprocal experience of growth in self-knowledge and in awareness of others has a powerful and positive effect on community cohesion. Such meetings produce many comments such as, "I never realised that …" and "now I understand why …" As the community members begin to understand themselves and one another more, the foundation stones for change are laid.

Since people cannot be expected to change their approach to life on the basis of nine weeks' work, however, the workshop can only be seen as the starting point for changes within a community. So workshop participants are encouraged to continue meeting by themselves after the last session is completed. These continued meetings enable participants to sustain the changes that they have decided to make in their lives and act as a support group. They enable people to compare and share their successes and failures and to renew their determination to do things differently in future – something made easier by sharing the experience with a group of similarly committed people.

How Stepping Stones motivates and mobilises men

- Preparation for Stepping Stones' work in a community involves participatory needs assessment and discussion with community leaders, resource persons and existing grassroots groups, thus creating prior interest in the process among influential men.

- By dividing participants into age and gender groups, the workshop respects cultural norms of dialogue on sexual health issues. This motivates participation by men.

- Facilitators of men's groups are always men of similar age, usually from the community where the workshop is being conducted.

- The groups themselves decide the venue and time for their meetings, ensuring the process is built around their convenience and commitments. This encourages men's regular attendance.

- The approach helps men deal explicitly with their own mortality, and prepare for the security of their families through will writing. This is empowering in that it allows men to feel valued and retain the status of head of the household even when dealing with death.

- The methodology is not restricted to a community context but can also be used in schools and colleges, as well as the 'shop floor' context of industries, mining and other workplace environments.

Positive changes that can happen after using Stepping Stones

Sixteen months after a Stepping Stones workshop had been conducted in a community in Uganda, each of the four separate groups involved was interviewed separately about the changes they perceived in the community. It was a useful cross-reference to see that each reported change was mentioned by at least two separate groups. Young men and young women reported that they now had a better sense of trust between them. Previously, each had been blaming the other group for spreading AIDS – now, however, members of both these groups described how they had realised that they had to work together to overcome the challenge.

Young men also reported that they were starting to visit and help people with HIV and their carers in the community. Whilst older women had been doing this anyway, the young men said that they had previously just ignored or even ridiculed such people. Now, however, they reported that they had decided to do something to help them.

Most of the groups (which had not existed prior to the workshop) had also continued to meet regularly over the ensuing months. This would appear to be another key ingredient to sustained change. The one group which did not continue to meet was the older men's group, leading to some reported problems.

Conclusions

Learning about something, especially something as frightening as HIV, rarely influences people sufficiently to change their actions in a sustainable manner. Stepping Stones offers women and men of all ages and backgrounds the possibility of feeling safe about exploring – and learning to take more control of – the most personal details of their lives. When people feel able to begin to address these issues, about which they have immediate felt concerns for themselves, they are also helping to challenge conventional attitudes about women's rights, about traditional gender roles and about their own behaviours. They also begin to meet their own sexual and reproductive health needs.

In this way, sex, death and gender can begin to become less taboo subjects and therefore less fearful, and the causes and consequences of gender conflict can begin to be tackled. Work in such areas will also decrease vulnerability to HIV transmission and enable it to be addressed as an extension of these other issues, rather than as an isolated and insurmountable problem which bears no relation to the rest of people's lives.

Source: ActionAid, 2000; Welbourn, 1999

Case Study: The School Without Walls: Sharing Knowledge and Skills with Community Groups (Southern Africa)

The tortoise knows how to embrace his wife.

West African proverb

Introduction

Since the beginning of the international response to HIV in 1986, there have been numerous 'training programmes' designed to transfer North American expertise to Africa. The common approach of these programmes is to 'trickle down' the knowledge of a small group of northern experts, through a 'training of trainers' mechanism, to a large group of African field workers. Meanwhile, many African organisations developed extraordinary skills and knowledge because they had to find ways of living with a very serious situation affecting them directly. However, little attention was paid to validating and disseminating this local knowledge. This issue was identified in 1993 by community-based organisations supported by the Southern African AIDS Training (SAT) Programme. In response, SAT launched an initiative called School Without Walls (SWW).

The School Without Walls combines 18 Southern African organisations active in specific areas of the response to HIV, who have committed themselves to transfer their knowledge and skills to emerging community groups. The SAT Programme provides assistance to facilitate this transfer. The SWW approach is based on learning by seeing and doing in real settings, using results-oriented training that emphasises 'how to do' rather than 'what to do'. The transfer of skills within the SWW is from organisation to organisation.

The conception of the School Without Walls

When the world first woke up to the reports of a potentially serious HIV epidemic in Africa, the understandable immediate reaction was to mobilise all available expertise to stop the spread of the virus. This was the origin of the 'war against AIDS', introduced by the first Director of the Global Programme on AIDS. Many things have since been learned about HIV, however. The virus does not present itself as the convenient object of war. It does not 'attack' people and communities but is part of people and communities. How big a part depends less on the nature of the virus than on the environment in which transmission occurs. Although the necessary condition for an HIV epidemic is the presence of HIV, the shape of the epidemic is determined by many other factors of social structure and organisation.

As Africans confronted the emerging HIV epidemics in the continent, two errors of the early international campaigns stand out prominently: The focus was on the crisis rather than on the response; and there was too much reliance on theoretical disease prevention models, ignoring the fact that societies living with the virus were already applying their local knowledge to dealing with the situation. In retrospect, it should have been recognised that people facing challenges to life and livelihood tend to work out solutions long before international experts even grasp the nature of the problems.

The Southern African AIDS Training Programme (SAT) was set up in 1990 with Canadian government support and started building partnerships with groups in Southern Africa who began to organise to meet the emerging needs generated by the HIV epidemic. Initially most took a narrow view of these needs and developed their response within restrictive margins. Some groups were active in health education, others

. . . people facing challenges to life and livelihood tend to work out solutions long before international experts even grasp the nature of the problems.

Throughout the 1990s, the HIV epidemic in Southern Africa expanded to unprecedented levels.

specialised in peer group activities among sex workers, some developed home care programmes and others confined their activities to supportive counselling. Some of the SAT partners did not explicitly include the response to HIV in their mandate. These were groups working for child welfare, groups who saw their main mandate as preventing domestic violence and groups lobbying for the legal rights of women or for human rights. Many of the groups were religious and mission based, reflecting the prominent role of the churches in providing health and social services in rural areas of Southern Africa.

Throughout the 1990s, the HIV epidemic in Southern Africa expanded to unprecedented levels. The groups and organisations trying to respond to the growing social and health needs came under pressure to expand their response, both in magnitude and in scope. Organisations that had started with the offer of specific prevention programmes had to integrate counselling and care in their services. Groups that had formed with a mandate to help victims of domestic violence were flooded by demands of women who were abused because of their HIV infection. Service organisations working for the protection of children from sexual abuse saw an increasing clientele of sexually abused orphans whose parents had died of AIDS. The social and AIDS service organisations had no difficulty knowing what needed to be done but faced the problem of not knowing how to do it. The issues that confronted them were new and there was little organisational experience in formulating an appropriate and functional response.

In 1993, a group of Southern African organisations met with SAT Programme staff and raised the following challenge: How can we access the expertise and skills developed by local groups who have found solutions to the problems we are facing every day? Clearly, these organisations did not want another series of lectures and workshops designed by experts. They did not need more 'AIDS awareness' or more generic 'programme management training'. They wanted facilitated access to local solutions developed by their peers. This was the birth of the School Without Walls. The event was a milestone in the SAT Programme philosophy as the word 'training' in its name changed its meaning from the transfer of expertise to Africa to address problems identified in North America to the validation and diffusion of African solutions to problems identified in Africa.

What is the School Without Walls?

Today, the School Without Walls is a loose network with 18 organisations at its core, each with a unique and specific experience in conducting activities relevant to the response to HIV in Southern Africa. The types of activities of the School Without Walls partner organisations are:

- Providing comprehensive HIV prevention, care and social support services;

- Addressing issues of HIV in the workplace through policy and peer education programmes;

- Providing counselling and palliative care services;

- Conducting programmes to prevent domestic violence and providing services for women and children who are victims of violence;

- Supporting peer action programmes for HIV prevention and care among female sex workers and other marginalised groups;

- Producing material for public education on HIV.

Through the School Without Walls, the organisations provide training in their specific areas of expertise with co-ordination and financial support from the SAT Programme. The training mandate extends to the whole of the Southern African region but is most involved in Zimbabwe, Zambia, Tanzania, Malawi and Mozambique. The methods of training include:

Structured study visits
Less experienced groups or organisations who want to introduce new programme areas visit more experienced organisations to observe their programmes in action. The visiting and host organisations are carefully matched to ensure the relevance of the concepts and skills to be transferred.

Organisational mentoring

Experienced organisations take on a mentoring role for new groups over a period of several weeks to several months. During this time, experienced staff of the mentoring organisation help design programmes, supervise and monitor the activities, and solve technical and administrative problems on the basis of need and demand. Mentoring often develops into long-term organisational relationships of mutual benefit to both parties.

Apprenticeships

Apprenticeships are usually organised in the context of mentoring relationships. They are an attachment of personnel for periods of one to four weeks to a well established programme, to gain practical experience in areas such as counselling, home care, managing of peer education programmes or providing services for victims of domestic and sexual violence.

Skills clinics

Skills clinics are practical group exercises usually lasting two to five days organised by the School Without Walls training organisations within their own working environment. They comprise personal coaching, group exercises and field visits. Skills clinics are a means for new organisations and for new personnel to rapidly acquire the basic knowledge about how to do what it is they have set themselves to do. The orientation of the clinics is towards basic project implementation skills in common areas of work.

Specialised skills clinics

Specialised skills clinics have a somewhat different objective. They are organised and hosted by one School Without Walls training organisation with a specific activity profile. The participants usually come from the entire region and may include other organisations with the same level of expertise in the subject. The skills clinics thereby function not only as a one-way transfer of know-how from trainer to trainee, but also as a forum to exchange programme experience and to find solutions to problems mutually encountered. Specialised skills clinics are organised on a variety of themes, such as domestic violence, child sexual abuse, counselling for survival skills among people living with HIV, home care, palliative care and bereavement counselling.

Thematic networks

Thematic networks are not strictly a method for capacity transfer but rather a mechanism of mutual support and learning for specialised organisations. The networks may be national or regional and often evolve from specialised skills clinics. Network members include all organisations with interest or activities in specific areas such as supportive counselling, home care and human rights advocacy. Although supported by the SAT Programme, the networks extend well beyond SAT and the School Without Walls and often include government representatives of the relevant ministries and programmes.

Cross networking

Cross networking is organised and directly managed by the SAT Programme using the School Without Walls structure. The purpose is to widen the goals and perspectives of organisations working in areas related to the response to HIV. For instance, a series of cross networking meetings organised by SAT brought together activists on gender equality, human rights activists and AIDS activists from several countries in Southern Africa. This allowed the different organisations to identify common areas of activity and interest. As a result, some AIDS and gender activist groups formed a common approach to address the issue of property rights for widows and achieved significant results in terms of public awareness and legal reform.

The School Without Walls programme and approach has become well established in Southern Africa. Institutional mentoring, site visits, apprenticeship exchanges and thematic networks are being organised well beyond the boundaries of the SAT Programme, supported by a large number of international donors. It has become a practical model of South–South collaboration and is a viable alternative to the trickling down of not necessarily appropriate theoretical knowledge to field workers via the sometimes very tenuous information chain of 'training of trainers'.

Source: Beatson and Decosas, 2000

Case Study: Integrating Sexual and Reproductive Health Programmes (Bangladesh)

In Bangladesh, the International Centre for Diarrhoeal Disease Research (ICDDR,B) and the Bangladesh Rural Advancement Committee (BRAC) joined forces to integrate sexual health interventions and education into existing rural health services. For economic and other reasons, the integration of HIV/AIDS activities into existing programmes offers a viable approach to controlling the pandemic. A narrowly focused HIV/AIDS programme may fail to mobilise the community for effective control and prevention and may even meet with opposition. Integrated programmes that deliver a wide range of services can be more effective and attract support from many segments of society. Another reason for including HIV/AIDS components in ongoing programmes is the need to ensure sustainability of prevention efforts.

The goal of the joint project was to improve the sexual and reproductive health of the rural poor in Bangladesh, especially women and adolescent girls. In an effort to reach this goal, the project undertook a number of steps that are needed to successfully integrate STI/HIV activities into existing health services. These included:

- Conducting a needs assessment (interviews and focus groups) within the community to identify the socio-cultural factors contributing to the need for sexual and reproductive health services among community members. This allowed the programme to explore:

  - myths, beliefs and taboos about sex and HIV/AIDS;

  - relationships between men and women;

  - knowledge, attitude and practices in HIV/AIDS prevention;

  - populations in need of services;

  - level of community interest in the programme;

  - types of services needed.

- Identifying and training community members interested in becoming peer educators and counsellors.

- Training community health workers to integrate sexual and reproductive health education into their work. The workers began to discuss sexual and reproductive health issues with their clients during their regular visits, regardless of the nature of the visit (i.e., birth attendants, pharmacists and traditional healers added sexual health education to their regular routine). Community members began to view the health providers as resources on sexual problems in addition to their existing roles.

- Creating educational materials based on the results of their needs assessment. The materials included picture stories containing information about physical development, reproduction, STIs and hygiene. The materials were used to train the health workers and peer educators.

- Conducting an evaluation of the integrated health services.

Through the project's efforts, 68 health workers and 1,890 community members were trained to integrate sexual and reproductive health services into their work. The trained personnel talked to hundreds of community members, providing them with the information and resources to deal with sexual health problems in addition to the regular services provided.

Source: UNAIDS, 2001a

Sexual health not only requires appropriate levels of knowledge about sexuality. It also requires the capacity to develop fully one's potential for sexual expression . . .

Case Study: Gender Differences in Sexual Health Promotion among Adolescents (Canada)

Sexual health not only requires appropriate levels of knowledge about sexuality. It also requires the capacity to develop fully one's potential for sexual expression (Blonna and Levitan, 2000). Such capacity is particularly important for adolescents and young adults as they begin to explore issues of sexuality and sexual activity. With sexual exploration comes the very real potential for unintended pregnancies as well as exposure to sexually transmitted infections (STIs), including HIV.

Many efforts have been undertaken to reduce the incidence of STIs and unintended pregnancies among adolescents. However, the types of healthy sexuality messages targeted at this population are often at odds with the way young men and women are socialised. For example, programmes for adolescents that place a significant emphasis on contraceptive choices for pregnancy prevention may have the effect of inadvertently shifting these messages from both males and females to an issue for females alone. Differing definitions of healthy sexuality and differences in areas of sexual interest between young men and women may also serve to reinforce traditional gender stereotypes and sex roles that portray females as passive and males as active sexual beings.

Since 1996, the community of Amherst in Nova Scotia, Canada, has been making efforts to help young people with this aspect of their lives through health promotion efforts targeted particularly at prevention of STIs and unintended pregnancy. During this time, the Amherst Association for Healthy Adolescent Sexuality (AAHAS), a voluntary non-profit organisation, has been conducting community education, largely through a campaign making use of local media, workshops for parents and continuing professional education, all directed at improving the sexual health of Amherst's adolescents. A health centre located at Amherst Regional High School (ARHS) has been established to provide educational and clinical services to students through a nurse-educator. These services include contraceptive and sexual health counselling and referral, and the provision of free condoms.

In order to assess the success of this programme, students at ARHS were asked to complete self-administered questionnaires in November 1996 and again in November 1999. They were asked about their sexual health knowledge, their attitudes towards various aspects of sexuality and their use of barrier protection and oral contraception. Questionnaires were administered in the classroom setting, supervised by teachers. Approximately 80 per cent of eligible students completed surveys in both survey years. The mean ages of students by gender were very similar, as were proportions of eligible males and females responding.

Some of the results of surveys were that:

- Sexual activity was similar in 1996 and in 1999 for males and was seen to decrease slightly in females.

- Sexual health knowledge scores increased in both age groups in each gender, both overall and in those who were sexually active. Absolute differences were similar for females, both overall and for those who were sexually active. Males who were sexually active had a smaller increase in knowledge than that seen in males overall.

- For males overall, attitudes towards condoms remained the same from 1996 to 1999, but the attitudes of sexually active males became less positive. Females in both groups showed more favourable attitudes.

- Females had significant increases in their perception of societal support for their use of condoms, while males indicated decreased perception of such support.

- Use of a condom at last intercourse increased significantly in females from 1996 to 1999, but was essentially unchanged in males.

- Females' use of oral contraception at last intercourse increased from 49 per cent to 58 per cent.

There was also an approximately 31 per cent reduction in the pregnancy rate in Amherst in 1998 attributable to the intervention effect.

The changes in young women's sexual health attitudes and behaviours, and in rates of pregnancy observed in association with this programme, are very encouraging. Young men, however, did not show much in the way of change over the three-year period. In fact, though males showed an increase in knowledge, changes in attitude towards condoms and perception of societal support for their use were essentially the same in both years, and attitudes to condoms in fact became less positive. This was reflected in the finding that males' condom use at last intercourse remained unchanged. Despite the efforts made to include both male and female students' needs in sexual health promotion messages in both school-based and community programmes, young women responded more favourably to these messages than young men. This finding is similar to those seen in other investigations (Gupta, Weiss and Mane, 1996).

Some authors suggest that such results may be related to differences in levels of maturity between adolescent males and females. Others argue that this is a reflection of a sexual double standard, whereby young women are socialised to accept a greater degree of responsibility for sexual and reproductive outcomes than their male counterparts (Blonna and Levitan,

The changes in young women's sexual health attitudes and behaviours, and in rates of pregnancy . . . are very encouraging.

Educational interventions which include role-play, question and answer sessions, and computer-based information and sexual health assessment tools have been found to be very useful among adolescents.

2000; Goma, 1996). It could also be the case that the community's health promotion efforts may not have sufficiently taken into account the needs of the young men it was attempting to reach. Efforts to reduce the spread of STIs, including HIV, as well as unintended pregnancies, must acknowledge the variability of high school aged individuals' sexual experiences in addition to the gender differences in sexual socialisation between young men and women. Additional sexual health promotion programming efforts in this community will need to take measures to ensure that young men feel a sense of 'buy in' with such efforts and do not feel as though they have been written out of the safer sex discourse.

Perhaps negative attitudes seen among the young men in this study are a reaction to a new sense of empowerment on the part of young women in Amherst. Culturally dominant ideas or gender stereotypes regarding sexual roles and responsibilities for high school aged individuals can present formidable challenges in the prevention of STIs, HIV and unintended pregnancies, and should be considered by those involved in such efforts.

Providing sexual health information to young people might be more useful if it also provided the means to change behaviours in the context of their own unique social and cultural frameworks. The decisions made by young people regarding prevention in the area of sexual health are often informed by social and cultural values that reflect the social context in which more general decisions regarding sexuality are made (Kowalewski et al., 1997). Several authors have pointed to the need to go beyond simply attempting to increase awareness of risks to sexual health. Reference also needs to be made to the numerous risks confronted by young people in the context of their daily lives (Schieman, 1998; Poppen and Reisen, 1997; Smith and Katner, 1995).

Educational interventions which include role-play, question and answer sessions, and computer-based information and sexual health assessment tools have been found to be very useful among adolescents. A number of authors call for interventions which allow both young men and women to act out and discuss inconsistencies between levels of perceived risk and imposed responsibility and actual risk behaviours. Others report that stereotypical sex roles will continue to undermine prevention efforts unless adolescents have access to resources and environmental supports to sustain such efforts (Rhodes et al., 1997; Rotheram-Borus et al., 1995; Stevenson et al., 1995). Issues of the context in which sexual risk behaviours occur need to be addressed, together with the impact of gender roles – including sex role stereotypying and the sexual double standard – on sexual risk-taking behaviours. Until then, many young people will continue to find themselves at enhanced risk of unintended pregnancies, STIs and HIV infection.

Source: Langille, Gahagan and Flowerdew, 2001

5. Tools and Resources

Gender Sensitivity Checklist

The following checklist is a component of the UNAIDS Resource Packet on Gender and AIDS. Its aim is to provide HIV/AIDS policy makers and educators with a tool to assess the gender sensitivity of their programmes and policies. It covers three areas: Development, Implementation and Organisational Structure.

Programme/policy development

Does your programme policy:

- [ ] Encourage community members, especially women and girls, to participate in the development planning process?

- [ ] Use innovative and non-traditional means to solicit the participation of community members, especially women and girls, in the development planning process? (For example, hold planning sessions where women usually gather, provide services to women so they can forgo their daily tasks in order to participate, etc.)

- [ ] Encourage community groups, especially women's groups, to participate in the development planning process?

- [ ] Encourage people living with HIV/AIDS (PLHA), especially women and girls, to participate in the development planning process?

- [ ] Include all participants, especially women and girls, in the development of programme/policy goals and objectives?

- [ ] Provide gender training for programme facilitators?

- [ ] Include facilitators who are members of the programme's target population?

- [ ] Include facilitators who are comfortable with discussing gender-sensitive issues?

☐ Tailor activities to the particular economic, political and cultural realities of participants?

☐ Tailor activities to address the power imbalances between women and men and between girls and boys?

☐ Include participatory activities (group activities, role playing, brainstorming, mapping, story telling, etc.)?

☐ Produce educational materials that promote positive representations of women, men, girls and boys, as well as PLHA?

☐ Occur at a time and place that is convenient to all participants, especially women and girls?

☐ Provide transportation for participants in an effort to encourage attendance?

☐ Provide child-care for participants during programme activities?

Programme/policy implementation

Does your programme/policy:

☐ Encourage community members, especially women and girls, to participate in peer education? (For example, leading segments of the workshop/discussions, demonstrating condom use, etc.)

☐ Encourage PLHA, especially women and girls, to participate in programme implementation?

☐ Provide access to information and knowledge about HIV/AIDS to all participants equally?

☐ Encourage discussion about socially assigned gender roles affecting women, men, adolescents and the elderly?

☐ Enable women and men, and girls and boys, to understand one another's needs?

☐ Attempt to ensure that women and men, and girls and boys, are listening to the needs of one another? (For example, have participants represent one another in role play, have participants summarise and repeat the issues raised in discussion, etc.)

☐ Encourage discussion of the various social factors, such as economics, politics and social structures, that put women or men more at risk for HIV/AIDS?

☐ Encourage discussion of the biological factors that put women or men more at risk for HIV/AIDS?

☐ Encourage discussion of how gender inequality affects HIV/AIDS prevention, transmission, treatment and care?

☐ Address the financial difficulties brought on by HIV/AIDS, which often disproportionately affect women and girls? (For example, laws which do not allow women to inherit land from their husbands, the need for widows to seek out new forms of income to support their families, the burden of health care costs which often become the responsibility of women, etc.)

☐ Encourage discussion of the power imbalance between women and men, girls and boys, and how these imbalances affect the transmission and prevention of HIV/AIDS? (For example, the difficulties women face in insisting that their partners use condoms, the ability to choose when and with whom to have sex, etc.)

☐ Encourage discussion of how empowerment of women and girls could help lessen their vulnerability to HIV/AIDS? (It is crucial to include men and boys in this discussion so they can participate and support their wives, sisters and mothers as opposed to becoming threatened by their empowerment.)

☐ Work to eliminate the power imbalance between women and men and between girls and boys?

☐ Address the issue of violence against women and girls?

☐ Provide opportunities for women and girls to become empowered through HIV/AIDS education? (For example, enhance the self-confidence of women and girls by encouraging them to attain new skills, take on more responsibilities as desired, become local leaders in health promotion, etc.)

☐ Encourage and acknowledge the support that women and girls can provide to one another.

☐ Encourage equal communication among participants about sexuality, sexual health and sex practices (dry sex, anal sex, sex with commercial sex workers, etc.)?

☐ Address the double standard that exists between men and women in relation to sexual activity? (For example, men being allowed to engage in sex outside of marriage while women are not, men being expected to have sexual experience before marriage while women are not, etc.)

☐ Address the issue of sexual abuse (rape, incest, etc.)?

☐ Address adolescent sexuality and the affect it may have on HIV/AIDS?

☐ Address the importance of equal access to education for both girls and boys?

☐ Address the sexual and reproductive health needs of children and adolescents?

☐ Facilitate awareness in adults of the sexual and reproductive health needs of children and adolescents?

☐ Encourage adults to address the sexual and reproductive health needs of children and adolescents?

☐ Provide demonstrations to all participants on how to use both the male and the female condoms and encourage all participants to practice their use?

☐ Encourage discussion about the possible difficulties associated with condom use experienced by both women and men?

☐ Address how HIV/AIDS affects how women and men make reproductive choices?

☐ Encourage the involvement of both women and men in family planning?

☐ Address how to avoid HIV transmission from mother to child (both before and during birth)?

☐ Address the need to improve the quality of health services for women and girls?

☐ Address the need to improve access to health services for women and girls (transportation, financial, etc.)?

☐ Address the various health care changes that occur over a lifetime and how these changes affect HIV/AIDS treatment and prevention? (For example, a women's health needs and HIV/AIDS susceptibility may change significantly as her body changes through adolescence, childbearing years and menopause.)

☐ Encourage men and boys to participate equally in HIV/AIDS prevention efforts?

☐ Encourage men and boys to help with domestic tasks as women's lives are impacted by HIV? (Greater assistance with domestic tasks may be needed if a mother, sister or wife becomes ill, if she has to care for infected loved ones, if she has to begin to generate the family income, etc.)

☐ Encourage men to become more involved in the care of their families?

Organisational structure

Does your organisation:

☐ Have stated policies that affirm a commitment to gender awareness (goals and objectives, mission statement, etc.)?

☐ Encourage and support participation among women and men in practices and activities? (For example, do both women and men have an opportunity to participate in discussions, to manage and develop programmes/projects, to hold advisory positions, to participate equally in planning and implementation of services, etc.)

☐ Monitor internal practices in an effort to identify areas that are not currently gender sensitive?

☐ Continually adapt internal practices in an effort to remain gender sensitive?

☐ Support gender awareness among staff? (For example, provide gender sensitivity training to staff members at all levels.)

☐ Have ideas of gender sensitivity formalised at all levels? (For example, include gender sensitive practices from entry level positions through top management level.)

☐ Employ both women and men?

☐ Provide women with access to a variety of positions at all employment levels?

☐ Pay women and men the same for equal work?

☐ Support the needs of employees, both women and men, with families? (For example, provide child-care facilities, allow employees to work flexible schedules, provide leave to care for loved ones, etc.)

☐ Provide both women and men with access to training activities and extension services to facilitate professional development?

Source: Bunch, 2001

Online Resources

AEGIS: *www.aegis.org/*
The largest HIV/AIDS website in the world, AEGIS contains a large, searchable database of news stories, newsletter articles, community materials and AIDS abstracts from journals and conferences.

AIDS.ORG: *www.aids.org*
AIDS.ORG (previously Immunet) is a non-profit organisation dedicated to harnessing the power of the Internet in the battle against HIV/AIDS.

AIDS and Africa: *www.aidsandafrica.com/*
The AIDS and Africa site offers comprehensive, up-to-date information on HIV/AIDS in Africa.

AIDS Clinical Trials Information Service (ACTIS): *www.actis.org/*
ACTIS provides quick and easy access to information on federally and privately funded clinical trials for adults and children in the United States.

Aidsmap: *www.aidsmap.com/*
Aidsmap is a massive compendium of news, treatments, services and literature. The site is produced by the National AIDS Manual (NAM Publications) in collaboration with the British HIV Association and St. Stephen AIDS Trust.

AmfAR: *www.amfar.org*
AmfAR is the United States' leading non-profit organisation dedicated to the support of HIV/AIDS research into prevention methods (including a vaccine), improved treatments and ultimately a cure.

AVERT: *www.avert.org/*
AVERT is a UK-based AIDS education and medical research charity that focuses on information about education to prevent infection with HIV, information for HIV-positive people and the latest news and statistics.

B.C. Centre for Excellence in HIV/AIDS:
cfeweb.hivnet.ubc.ca/pages/main/conmain.html
B.C. Centre for Excellence in HIV/AIDS (British Columbia, Canada) provides education to health care providers, conducts natural history and observational studies, develops innovative laboratory tests and carries out clinical trials.

Canadian Aboriginal AIDS Network Inc. (CAAN):
www.caan.ca/
CAAN is a non-profit coalition of individuals and organisations which provides leadership, support and advocacy for Aboriginal people living with and affected by HIV/AIDS, regardless of where they reside.

Canadian Association for HIV Research:
www.cahr-acrv.ca/portail.htm
The Canadian Association for HIV Research aims to serve as a professional association for all individuals in Canada interested in research on HIV/AIDS and to foster collaboration between Canadian scientists and investigators.

Canadian Health Coalition: *www.healthcoalition.ca*
The Canadian Health Coalition is dedicated to preserving and enhancing Canada's public health system for the benefit of all Canadians.

Canadian HIV/AIDS Clearinghouse:
www.clearinghouse.cpha.ca/
The Canadian HIV/AIDS Clearinghouse provides information on HIV/AIDS prevention, care and support to health and education professionals, AIDS Service Organisations, health information resource centres, governments and others.

Canadian HIV Trials Network (CTN):
www.hivnet.ubc.ca/ctn.html
CTN is a partnership committed to developing treatments, vaccines and a cure for HIV disease and AIDS, through the conduct of scientifically sound and ethical clinical trials.

Canadian Institutes for Health Research (CIHR):
www.cihr.ca/index.shtml
CIHR is Canada's federal agency for health research and offers access to numerous documents on research in the area of HIV/AIDS.

Canadian Women's Health Network: *cwhn.ca*
The Canadian Women's Health Network shares information, resources and strategies, and builds links to improve women's health

Canadian Working Group on HIV and Rehabilitation (CWGHR): *www.hivandrehab.ca*
CWGHR is a national, autonomous, multi-sectoral and multidisciplinary working group which facilitates a national, co-ordinated response to emerging needs in rehabilitation in the context of HIV.

Centers for Disease Control & Prevention (CDC) National Prevention Information Network: *www.cdcnpin.org/*
The CDC National Prevention Information Network is an information service of the national US centre for HIV, STI and TB prevention.

Centres of Excellence for Women's Health (Canada):
  British Columbia Centre of Excellence for Women's Health
  www.bccewh.bc.ca
  Le Centre d'excellence pour la santé des femmes, Consortium Université de Montréal:
  www.cesaf.umontreal.ca
  Maritime Centre of Excellence for Women's Health:

www.medicine.dal.ca/mcewh
National Network on Environments and Women's Health
(NNEWH): *www.yorku.ca/nnewh/*
Prairie Women's Health Centre of Excellence:
www.pwhce.ca
These five centres of excellence for women's health have as
their mission to improve the health of women by fostering collaboration on innovative, multi-disciplinary research endeav-
ours and action-oriented approaches to women's health initiatives, women-centred programmes and health policy.

Commonwealth Secretariat: *www.thecommonwealth.org/gender*
The Commonwealth is a leading international voice on the
promotion of gender equality. This site of the Commonwealth's Gender and Youth Affairs Division includes information on government mandates and downloadable publications.
(See also *www.youngcommonwealth.org* and *www.thecommon-
wealth.org*).

Community AIDS Treatment Information Exchange (CATIE):
www.catie.ca/aboutcatie.html
CATIE is a national, non-profit organisation committed to
improving the health and quality of life of all Canadians living
with HIV/AIDS.

Elizabeth Glaser Pediatric AIDS Foundation (EGPAF):
www.pedaids.org/
EGPAF is a worldwide non-profit organisation dedicated to
identifying, funding and conducting pediatric HIV/AIDS
research, as well as other serious and life-threatening diseases
involving children.

European AIDS Treatment Group (EATG): *www.eatg.org/*
EATG is a pan-European organisation committed to support-
ing HIV treatment activism and people living with HIV and
AIDS across Europe.

Family Health International (FHI):
www.fhi.org/en/aids/naids.html
FHI has pioneered ways to curtail the spread of HIV/AIDS.
Many of the HIV prevention best practices in use today have
emerged from FHI's work in more than 60 countries.

Global Health Council: *www.globalhealthcouncil.org/*
The Global Health Council is the world's largest membership alliance dedicated to improving health worldwide.

Health Canada: *www.hc-sc.gc.ca/hppb/hiv_aids/*
Health Canada's website on HIV/AIDS.

HIV and AIDS Legal Clinic Ontario (HALCO): *www.halco.org/body.htm*
HALCO is a not-for-profit, community-based legal clinic serving low-income people with HIV/AIDS in Ontario, Canada.

HIV and Hepatitis.com: *www.hivandhepatitis.com/html/hiv_aids.html*
HIV and Hepatitis.com is a quality online publication that provides practical, reliable information about treatment and experimental vaccine options for HIV and hepatitis.

HIV InSite: *hivinsite.ucsf.edu/*
HIV InSite is a gateway to in-depth information about particular aspects of HIV/AIDS. It is a project of the University of California San Francisco (UCSF) Positive Health Programme at San Francisco General Hospital Medical Centre and the UCSF Centre for AIDS Prevention Studies, which are programmes of the UCSF AIDS Research Institute.

Immunodeficiency Clinic, Toronto Hospital, Ontario, Canada: *www.tthhivclinic.com/index.html*
The Immunodeficiency Clinic of the Toronto Hospital in Ontario, Canada – part of the University Health Network – provides services for people with HIV/AIDS.

International AIDS Economic Network (IAEN): *www.iaen.org/*
IAEN provides data, tools and analysis on the economics of HIV/AIDS prevention and treatment in developing countries for compassionate, cost-effective responses to the global epidemic.

International AIDS Vaccine Initiative (IAVI): *www.iavi.org/*
IAVI is a global, non-profit organisation working to speed the development and distribution of preventive AIDS vaccines, which it sees as the world's best hope for ending the AIDS epidemic.

International Association of Physicians in AIDS Care (IAPAC): *www.iapac.org*
IAPAC is a non-profit association of more than 6,800 physicians and other healthcare professionals in 43 countries. IAPAC's educational services aim to expand access to cutting-edge clinical management information related to HIV and associated health complications.

International Labour Organization (ILO): *www.ilo.org/public/english/protection/trav/aids/index.htm*
This site contains information from the ILO on HIV/AIDS and the world of work.

Johns Hopkins AIDS Service: *www.hopkins-aids.edu*
The Johns Hopkins AIDS Service is provided as a resource for physicians and other healthcare professionals providing care and treatment to patients with HIV/AIDS.

Journal of the American Medical Association (JAMA) HIV/AIDS Information Centre:
www.ama-assn.org/special/hiv/
The JAMA HIV/AIDS Information Centre is designed as a resource for physicians and other health professionals. The site is produced and maintained by JAMA editors and staff under the direction of an editorial review board of leading HIV/AIDS authorities.

MAP Network: *www.cdpc.com/map.htm*
To highlight the 15th year of the pandemic, a worldwide network to monitor the AIDS pandemic (MAP) was launched on December 1, 1996. The MAP Network publishes reports regarding the status and trends of HIV/AIDS/STI epidemics around the world.

National AIDS Treatment Advocacy Project (NATAP): *www.natap.org/*
NATAP is a non-profit organisation based in the United States dedicated to educating communities affected by HIV on the latest treatments and advocating on treatment and policy issues for people with HIV.

New York Times:
www.nytimes.com/library/national/science/aids-index.html
This *New York Times* site contains coverage of the AIDS

pandemic from the beginning to the present and provides an excellent historical overview by Sean Gallagher.

Ontario HIV Treatment Network (OHTN): *www.ohtn.on.ca/*
OHTN ensures excellence in the care and treatment of people living with HIV in Ontario, Canada, while respecting the rights of individuals to confidentiality and privacy.

Project Inform: *www.projinf.org/*
Project Inform is a national non-profit, community-based organisation based in the USA working to end the AIDS epidemic. It has earned an international reputation as a vocal, active and effective advocate for the HIV/AIDS community it serves.

Red Ribbon: *www.redribbon.co.za/*
Red Ribbon is an African site dedicated to disseminating information about HIV/AIDS in the belief that information is an important tool with which to fight the disease.

Southern Africa AIDS Information Dissemination Service (SAfAIDS): *www.safaids.org.zw/*
SAfAIDS is a regional HIV/AIDS information dissemination service based in Zimbabwe that promotes, informs and supports appropriate responses to the epidemic in the fields of HIV prevention, care, support, long-term planning, and coping with the impact of AIDS.

UNAIDS: *www.unaids.org/*
UNAIDS leads, strengthens and supports an expanded response aimed at preventing the transmission of HIV, providing care and support, reducing the vulnerability of individuals and communities to HIV/AIDS, and alleviating the impact of the epidemic.

US Food and Drug Administration (FDA):
www.fda.oashi/aids/hiv.html
This site contains information regarding the FDA's HIV/AIDS Programme.

US National Institute of Allergy and Infectious Diseases (NIAID):
www.niaid.nih.gov/newsroom/focuson/hiv00/default.htm
NIAID provides support for research aimed at developing

better ways to diagnose, treat and prevent infectious, immuno-logic and allergic diseases.

World Health Organization (WHO):
www.who.int/health-topics/hiv.htm
This site contains information regarding the WHO initiative on HIV/AIDS and sexually transmitted infections, surveil-lance and response, WHO publications and its programmes.

YouthCO: *www.youthco.org/youthco.htm*
YouthCO is a Canadian AIDS service organisation working to meet the needs of both HIV-positive and HIV-negative youth.

List of Acronyms

AAHAS	Amherst Association for Healthy Adolescent Sexuality, Canada
AIDS	Acquired ImmunoDeficiency Syndrome
ARHS	Amherst Regional High School, Canada
BRAC	Bangladesh Rural Advancement Committee
CARICOM	The Caribbean Community
CEDAW	Convention on the Elimination of all forms of Discrimination Against Women
CGIAR	Consultative Group on International Agricultural Research
CHOGM	Commonwealth Heads of Government Meeting
CIHR	Canadian Institutes of Health Research
FAO	Food and Agriculture Organization
GIAAFS	Global Initiative on HIV/AIDS, Agriculture and Food Security
GMS	Gender Management System
HIV	Human Immunodeficiency Virus
ICDDR	International Centre for Diarrhoeal Disease Research
ICPD	International Conference on Population and Development (Cairo, 1994)
IDRC	International Development Research Centre
ICRW	International Center for Research on Women
ILO	International Labour Organization
IDU	Injection drug use
IPAA	International Partnership on AIDS in Africa
KIT	Royal Tropical Institute, The Netherlands
MTCT	Mother-to-child transmission
NACP	National AIDS Co-ordination Programme, Zimbabwe
NGO	Non-governmental organisation
OHCHR	Office of the High Commissioner for Human Rights
PFA	Beijing Platform for Action
PoA	Programme of Action of the ICPD
PSI	Population Services International

PTCT	Parent-to-child transmission
PLHA	People living with HIV/AIDS
SADC:	Southern African Development Community
SAfAIDS	Southern Africa AIDS Information Dissemination
SAT	Southern African AIDS Training Programme
STI	Sexually transmitted infection
SWW	School Without Walls
UNAIDS	Joint United Nations programme on HIV/AIDS
UNDCP	United Nations Office for Drug Control and Crime Prevention
UNDP	United Nations Development Programme
UNDPI	United Nations Department of Public Information
UNESCO	United Nations Educational, Scientific and Cultural Organization
UNICEF	United Nations Children's Fund
UNIFEM	United Nations Development Fund for Women
UNFPA	United Nations Population Fund
VCT	Voluntary Counselling and Testing
WHO	World Health Organization

Bibliography

Abamu, Frank (2002). 'Global Initiative on HIV/AIDS, Agriculture and Food Security'. Paper presented to the Feasibility Design Workshop on Gender and HIV/AIDS: Putting the Pieces Together, Maritime Centre of Excellence for Women's Health and Commonwealth Secretariat, Halifax, Nova Scotia, Canada, 16–18 January.

ActionAid (2000). *Safe Crossings: The Stepping Stones Approach to Involving Men in the Prevention of Violence and HIV Transmission*. London: ActionAid.

Alben, Anita and Lorna Guinness (2000). *Socio-Economic Impact of HIV/AIDS in Africa*, ADF, Joint United Nations Programme on HIV/AIDS (UNAIDS).

Albertyn, Cathi (2000). 'Prevention, Treatment and Care in the Context of Human Rights'. Paper presented to the UN Expert Group Meeting on Gender and HIV/AIDS, Windhoek, Namibia, 13–17 November.

Albert, Terry and Gregory Williams, with the collaboration of Barbara Legowski and Dr. Robert Remis (1998). *The Economic Burden of HIV/AIDS in Canada*, CPRN Study No. H02, Renouf Publishing.

Alexander, P. (1998). 'Prostitutes are being scapegoated for heterosexual AIDS'. In F. Delacsote and P. Alexander (eds). *Sex work: Writings by women in the sex industry*. London: Virago.

All India Institute of Hygiene and Public Health (1997). 'A Dream, a Pledge, a Fulfilment'. Annual Report. New Delhi, India.

Bayefsky, Anna F. (1994). 'General Approaches to Domestic Application of International Law'. In Rebecca Cook (ed.). *Human Rights of Women: National and International Perspectives*. Philadelphia: University of Pennsylvania Press.

Beatson, Ros and Josef Decosas (2000). 'The School Without Walls: A mechanism for the transfer of local knowledge for HIV programming in Southern Africa'. Paper presented by Felicitas Chiganze, Deputy Director, Southern African AIDS Training Programme, Harare, Zimbabwe at the Conference 'HIV/AIDS Programming in Developing Countries: Canada's Contribution'; Toronto, Canada, 1–2 June.

Blonna, R. and J. Levitan (2000). *Healthy Sexuality*. Colorado: Morton Publishing Company.

Bunch, Megan (2001). 'Gender Sensitivity Checklist'. In *UNAIDS*

Resource Packet on Gender & AIDS. Los Altos: Sociometrics.

Canadian Aids Society (Spring 2000), 'Women and HIV/AIDS', AIDS Awareness Campaign.

Canadian Woman Studies (2001). *Women and HIV/AIDS.* CWS/CF Vol. 21, No. 2. Summer/Fall.

Chinkin, Christine (2001). *Gender Mainstreaming in Legal and Constitutional Affairs.* London: Commonwealth Secretariat.

Commission on the Status of Women (2001). 'Agreed conclusions on women, the girl child and HIV/AIDS'. 45th Session of the UN CSW. New York: United Nations.

Commonwealth Secretariat (1998). *Youth Empowerment in the New Millennium: A Summary of the Commonwealth Plan of Action for Youth Empowerment.* London: Commonwealth Secretariat.

—— (1999a). *Gender and Health: Curriculum Outlines.* London: Commonwealth Secretariat.

—— (1999b). *Gender Management System Handbook.* London: Commonwealth Secretariat.

—— (1999c). *Gender Management Systems in the Health Sector.* Report of a Commonwealth Workshop, Halifax, Nova Scotia, Canada, 29 September–2 October.

—— (2001). 'A Multi-Sectoral Approach to Combating HIV/AIDS in Commonwealth Countries'. Report of a Commonwealth Think Tank Meeting, 19–20 June.

—— (2002). 'Gender Mainstreaming in HIV/AIDS: The Case for a Multisectoral Approach'. *Gender Dimensions in HIV/AIDS: A Commonwealth Approach*, Paper 1.

—— and Healthlink Worldwide (2001). *Gender and Relationships: A Practical Action Kit for Young People.* London: Commonwealth Secretariat.

Connor E.M., R.S. Sperling, R. Gelber et al. (1994). 'Reduction of Maternal-infant Transmission of Human Immunodeficiency Virus Type 1 with Zidovudine Treatment. Pediatric AIDS Clinical Trials Group Protocol 076 Study Group'. In *New England Journal of Medicine*, 331:1173–80.

Davidson, J. (1998). *Prostitution, Power and Freedom.* Ann Arbor: University of Michigan Press.

De Bruyn, Maria (2000). 'Gender, adolescents and the HIV/AIDS epidemic: The need for comprehensive sexual and reproductive health responses'. Paper presented to the UN Expert Group Meeting on Gender and HIV/AIDS, Windhoek, Namibia, 13–17 November.

DeYoung, Karen (2001). 'A Deadly Stigma in the Caribbean: As

AIDS Rate Soars, Infected are Shunned'. In *The Washington Post*, 19 July.

Dodds, Colin, Ronald Colman, Carol Amaratunga and Jeff Wilson (2001). 'The Economic Cost of HIV/AIDS in Canada'. Paper prepared for the Commonwealth Secretariat/Maritime Centre of Excellence for Women's Health co-publication.

Epstein, Daniel (2001). 'Confronting AIDS in the Caribbean: Major New Efforts Underway'. In *Perspectives in Health*, Vol. 6, No. 1. Washington DC: Pan American Health Organization (PAHO).

Family Health International (2001a). 'HIV Interventions with Youth'. State of the Art Briefs on HIV/AIDS. www.fhi.org/en/aids/impact/briefs/youth.html 24 January 2002.

—— (2001b). 'HIV Interventions with Men who have Sex with Men'. State of the Art Briefs on HIV/AIDS. www.fhi.org/en/aids/impact/briefs/msm.html 24 January 2002.

Farmer, Paul (1999). *Infections and Inequalities: The Modern Plagues*. Berkeley: The University of California Press.

Forbes J, D.R. Burdge and D. Money (1997). 'Pregnancy Outcome in HIV-infected Women in British Columbia: The Impact of Antiretroviral Therapy on Maternal-infant HIV Transmission'. In *Canadian Journal of Infectious Diseases*, March/April, Vol. 8:31A.

Forster, Jebbeh (2002). 'HIV/AIDS: A Strategy for Sierra Leone'. In Rawwida Baksh-Soodeen and Linda Etchart (eds). *Women and Men in Partnership for Post-Conflict Reconstruction: Report of the Sierra Leone National Consultation*, Freetown, Sierra Leone, 21–24 May 2001. London: Commonwealth Secretariat.

Gorna, R. (1996). *Vamps, Virgins and Victims*. London: Cassell.

Gómez, Adriana and Deborah Meacham, eds. (1998). 'Women, Vulnerability and HIV/AIDS: A Human Rights Perspective'. In *Women's Health Collection*/3. Chile: Latin American and Caribbean Women's Health Network.

Gould, Michelle and Amiram Gafni. 'Needle Exchange Programme and Economic Evaluation of a Local Experience'. In *Canadian Medical Association Journal*, No. 157.

Greaves, Lorraine, et al. (2000). *Sex, Gender and Women's Health*. Vancouver: Canadian Institutes of Health Research.

Gupta, Geeta Rao (2000a). 'Gender, Sexuality, and HIV/AIDS: The What, the Why, and the How', Plenary Address, XIII International AIDS Conference, Durban, South Africa, 12 July.

—— (2000b). 'Approaches for Empowering Women in the HIV/AIDS Pandemic: A Gender Perspective', Paper presented to the UN Expert Group Meeting on Gender and HIV/AIDS, Windhoek, Namibia, 13–17 November.

—— (2002). 'How men's power over women fuels the HIV epidemic'. In GENDER-AIDS, 31 January. Email: gender-aids@healthdev.net.

——, Ellen Weiss and Purnima Mane (1996). 'Talking About Sex: A Prerequisite for AIDS Prevention'. In Lynellen D. Long and E. Maxine Ankrah (eds). *Women's experiences with HIV/AIDS*. New York: Columbia University Press.

——, Ellen Weiss and Daniel Whelan (1996). 'Women and AIDS: Building a new HIV prevention strategy'. In Jonathan Mann and Daniel Tarantola (eds). *AIDS in the World II: Global Dimensions, Social Roots and Responses*. New York/Oxford: Oxford University Press.

Hamblin, Julie (1992). 'People Living with HIV: The Law, Ethics and Discrimination'. UNDP HIV and Development Programme Issues Paper No. 4. Paper prepared as a Plenary Presentation to the 2nd International Congress on AIDS in Asia and the Pacific, New Delhi, 8–12 November.

Hamblin, Julie and Elizabeth Reid (1991). 'Women, the HIV Epidemic and Human Rights: A Tragic Imperative'. UNDP HIV and Development Programme Issues Paper No. 8. Paper prepared for the International Workshop on 'AIDS: A Question of Rights and Humanity', International Court of Justice, The Hague.

Hancock (1998). *Shades of Grey: A Preliminary Overview of the Sex Trade Industry in London*. Report prepared for the Sex Trade Task Force, London, Ontario, Canada.

Hanvelt, Robin A., et al. (1994). 'Indirect Costs of HIV/AIDS Mortality in Canada'. In *AIDS* 8 (10).

Health Canada (2000a). *Gender-based Analysis Policy*. Ottawa: Health Canada.

—— (2000b). *HIV/AIDS EPI Update*. www.hc-sc.ca/hpb/lcdc/bah/epi/ahcan_e.html

—— (2000c). *HIV and AIDS in Canada: Surveillance Report to June 30, 2000*, Table 4C. Division of HIV/AIDS Surveillance, Bureau of HIV/AIDS, STD and TB, LCDC, HPB, Health Canada.

—— (2000d). *Perinatal Transmission of HIV*. HIV/AIDS Epi Updates, Bureau of HIV/AIDS, STD and TB, LCDC, HPB, Health Canada.

—— (2000e). HIV and AIDS in Canada: Surveillance Report to December 31,1999. Division of HIV/AIDS Surveillance, Bureau of HIV/AIDS, STD and TB, LCDC, HPB, Health Canada.

Health Canada's GBA Initiative (2001). *Moving Towards Equality: A Guide to Recognising and Eliminating Gender Bias in Health*. Ottawa: Health Canada.

Hellinger, Fred (1993). 'The Lifetime Cost of Treating a Person with HIV'. In *Journal of the American Medical Association*, 28 July, Vol. 270, no. 4.

Human Rights Watch (2001a). 'UN AIDS Conference Whitewash: US, Vatican, Egypt Undermining Frank Language in Conference Document'. Press release, New York, 20 June.

—— (2001b). 'AIDS and Human Rights: A Call for Action'. Press release, New York, 26 June.

International Labour Organization (2001). *An ILO Code of Practice on HIV/AIDS and the World of Work*. Geneva: ILO.

Iwere, Ngozi (2000). 'Community-level Interventions against HIV/AIDS from a Gender Perspective'. Paper presented to the UN Expert Group Meeting on Gender and HIV/AIDS, Windhoek, Namibia, 13–17 November.

Jackson, Lois (2001). 'HIV Prevention Programmes and Female Prostitutes: The Canadian Context'. Paper prepared for the Commonwealth Secretariat/Maritime Centre of Excellence for Women's Health co-publication.

——, A. Highcrest, and R. Coates (1992). 'Varied potential risks of HIV infection among female prostitutes'. In *Social Science & Medicine*, 35(3): 281–86.

—— and C. Hood (in press). 'Men's leisure, women's work: Female prostitutes and the double standard of North American HIV public health policies'. In Anderson and Lawrence (eds). *Gender Issues in Work and Leisure*.

Johnson, Tina (2001). 'Fatal Inequality: Women's Human Rights and the AIDS Crisis'. Course paper, Columbia University, April. Mimeograph.

Kerrigan, Deanna, Steve Mobley, Naomi Rutenberg, Andrew Fisher and Ellen Weiss (2000). *The Female Condom: Dynamics of Use in Urban Zimbabwe*. Washington: Horizons, The Population Council.

KIT, SAfAIDS and WHO (1995). *Facing the Challenges of HIV/AIDS/STDs: A Gender Response*. The Netherlands: Royal Tropical Institute (KIT).

Kowalewski, M.R., K.D. Henson and D. Longshore (1997). 'Rethinking perceived risk and health behaviour: A critical review of HIV prevention research'. In *Health Education Behavior*, 24: 313–325.

Kristoffersson, Ulf (2000). 'HIV/AIDS as a human security issue: A gender perspective'. Paper presented to the UN Expert Group Meeting on Gender and HIV/AIDS, Windhoek, Namibia, 13–17 November.

Kumar, Nikki, June Larkin and Claudia Mitchell (2001). 'Gender, Youth and HIV Risk'. In *Canadian Woman Studies*, Vol. 21, No. 2, Summer/Fall.

Langille, Donald B., Jacqueline Gahagan and Gordon Flowerdew (2001). 'Gender Differences in Results of a Programme to Promote the Sexual Health of High School Students in Nova Scotia'. Paper prepared for the Commonwealth Secretariat/Maritime Centre of Excellence for Women's Health co-publication.

Lapointe, N. (1998). 'Antiretroviral Therapy in Pregnant Women (CPARG): Access and Outcome (1995–1997) and the Experience of Transmission of HIV in Treated Pregnant Women at Ste. Justine's Clinic, Quebec'. In *Proceedings of a Scientific Meeting to Review the Vertical Transmission of HIV in Canada*, June.

Leonard, Lynne, Jacqueline Gahagan, Maryanne Doherty and Catherine Hankins (2001). 'HIV Counselling and Testing Among Pregnant Women in Canada: Best Practices'. Paper prepared for the Commonwealth Secretariat/Maritime Centre of Excellence for Women's Health co-publication.

Lerner, Sharon (2001). 'Product to protect women from HIV is elusive'. In *The New York Times*, 3 July.

Linkages (2001). 'Breastfeeding and HIV/AIDS: Frequently Asked Questions'. FAQ Sheet 1, May.

Loewenson, Rene and Alan Whiteside (2001). 'HIV/AIDS: Implications for Policy Reduction'. Background paper prepared for UNDP for the UNGASS on HIV/AIDS, 25–27 June. New York: UNDP.

Lomayani, Irene (2002). 'The Challenges of Confronting Gender and HIV/AIDS in Africa'. Paper presented to the Feasibility Design Workshop on Gender and HIV/AIDS: Putting the Pieces Together, Maritime Centre of Excellence for Women's Health and Commonwealth Secretariat, Halifax, Nova Scotia, Canada, 16–18 January.

Loppie, Charlotte and Jacqueline Gahagan (2001). 'Stacked Against Us: HIV/AIDS Statistics and Women'. In *Canadian Woman Studies*, Vol. 21, No. 2, Summer/Fall.

Machel, Graça (2000). 'The Impact of Armed Conflict on Children: A critical review of progress made and obstacles encountered in increasing protection for war-affected children'. Paper prepared for the International Conference on War-Affected Children, Winnipeg, Canada, September. http://www.unifem.undp.org/machelrep.html January 22, 2000.

—— (2001). 'Conflict fuels HIV/AIDS Crisis', in *Shaan: IPS Magazine on Gender and Human Rights*, Special issue for UN Special

Session on HIV/AIDS, New York, 25–27 June. Italy: Inter Press Service.

Mann, Jonathan and Daniel Tarantola, eds. (1996). *AIDS in the World II: Global Dimensions, Social Roots and Responses*. New York/Oxford: Oxford University Press.

Maritime Centre of Excellence for Women's Health (1998). 'Caregivers' Support Needs: Insights from the Experiences of Women Providing Care in Rural Nova Scotia'. In *Moving Towards Women's Health*, No. 1, November.

Matlin, Stephen and Nancy Spence (2000). 'The AIDS Pandemic and its Gender Implications'. Paper presented to the UN Expert Group Meeting on Gender and HIV/AIDS, Windhoek, Namibia, 13–17 November.

McGregor, Elizabeth and Fabiola Bazo (2001). *Gender Mainstreaming in Science and Technology*. London: Commonwealth Secretariat.

Millson, P., A. Moses, T. Myers, L. Calzavara, N. Degani, C. Chapman, C. Major and E. Wallace (2001). 'Gender, Injection Drug Use, and HIV Risk in Ontario, Canada'. Paper prepared for the Commonwealth Secretariat/Maritime Centre of Excellence for Women's Health co-publication.

Mzaidume, Zodwa, Catherine Campbell and Brian Williams (2000). 'Community-led HIV prevention by southern African sex workers'. In *Research for Sex Work* 3, June.

Nath, Madhu Bala (2001a). *From Tragedy to Hope: Men, women and the AIDS epidemic*. London: Commonwealth Secretariat.

—— (2001b). *Gender, HIV and Human Rights: A Training Manual*. New York: UNIFEM.

—— (2001c). *Gender and HIV/AIDS: Issues for the Commonwealth Secretariat*. London: Commonwealth Secretariat.

Obaid, Thoraya (2001). 'Africa is ground zero in fight against AIDS'. Op. Ed. in the *Boston Globe*, 22 June. 10 February 2002. http://www.boston.com/dailyglobe2/173/oped/Africa_is_ground_zero_in_fight_against_AIDS+.shtml

OHCHR and UNAIDS (1996). *HIV/AIDS and Human Rights: International Guidelines*. Geneva: OHCHR and UNAIDS.

Poppen P.J. and C.A. Reisen (1997). 'Perception of risk and sexual self-protective behavior: a methodological critique'. In *AIDS Education Preview*, 9: 373–390.

Ramjee, Gita, Eleanor Gouws, Amy Andrews, Landon Myer and Amy E. Weber (2001). 'Acceptability of a Vaginal Microbicide Among South African Men'. In *International Family Planning Perspectives*, Vol. 27, No. 4, December.

Rhodes F. M. Fishbein and J. Reis (1997). 'Using behavioral theory in computer-based health promotion and appraisal'. In *Health Education and Behavior*, 24: 20–34.

Rivers, Kim and Peter Aggleton (1999a). *Adolescent Sexuality, Gender and the HIV Epidemic*. New York: UNDP HIV and Development Programme.

—— (1999b). *Men and the HIV Epidemic, Gender and the HIV Epidemic*. New York: UNDP HIV and Development Programme.

Rose, Devin (2001). 'Distant hope: Activists are working to make American women see not just the violence against other women worldwide, but also that they can do something about it'. In *Chicago Tribune*, 4 July.

Rotheram-Borus M. J, K. A. Mahler and M. Rosario (1995). 'AIDS Prevention with adolescents'. In *AIDS Education Preview*, 7: 320–336.

Schieman S. (1998). 'Gender and AIDS-related psychosocial processes: A study of perceived susceptibility, social distance, and homophobia'. In *AIDS Education Preview*, 10: 264–277.

Seidlin, M. K. Krasinski, D. Bebenroth, V. Itri, A. M. Paolino and F. Valentine (1988). 'Prevalence of HIV infection in New York call girls'. In *Journal of Acquired Immune Deficiency Syndromes*, 1: 150–154.

Shahabudin, Sharifah H. (2000). 'Strategies of civil society to address AIDS in Asia: Emphasis on the sex sector'. Paper presented to the UN Expert Group Meeting on Gender and HIV/AIDS, Windhoek, Namibia, 13–17 November.

—— (2001). 'Women, the girl child and HIV/AIDS'. Written statement submitted to the 45th Session of the United Nations Commission on the Status of Women, New York, 6–16 March.

Shames, Stephen (2000). 'Uganda's brave fight against poverty and AIDS'. In *Choices: The Human Development Magazine*. New York: UNDP.

Ship, Susan Judith and Laura Norton (2001). 'HIV/AIDS and Aboriginal Women in Canada: A Case Study'. Paper prepared for the Commonwealth Secretariat/Maritime Centre of Excellence for Women's Health co-publication.

Smith, M. U. and H. P. Katner (1995). 'Quasi-experimental evaluation of three AIDS prevention activities for maintaining knowledge, improving attitudes, and changing risk behaviors of high school seniors'. In *AIDS Education Preview*, 7: 391–402.

Southern African AIDS Training Programme (2001). *Mainstreaming Gender in the Response to AIDS in Southern Africa: A Guide for the Integration of Gender Issues into the Work of AIDS Service Organisations*. Zimbabwe: SAT Programme.

Standing, Hilary (1998). 'Background paper in Health Systems Development prepared for the 12th Commonwealth Health Ministers Meeting, Nov. 1998'. In *Gender and Health Training Materials*. London: Commonwealth Secretariat.

Stevenson H.C., G.K. McKee and L. Josar (1995). 'Culturally sensitive AIDS education and perceived AIDS risk knowledge: Reaching the "know-it-all" teenager'. In *AIDS Education Preview*, 7:134–144.

Sy, Elhadj (2001). 'Women, the girl child and HIV/AIDS'. Written statement submitted to the 45th Session of the UN Commission on the Status of Women, New York, 6–16 March.

Tlou, Sheila Dinotshe (2000). 'Empowering Older Women in AIDS Prevention'. Paper presented to the UN Expert Group Meeting on Gender and HIV/AIDS, Windhoek, Namibia, 13–17 November.

—— (2001). 'Women, the Girl Child and HIV/AIDS'. Paper presented to a panel held at the UN Commission on the Status of Women, March 8.

Tolson, Margreth and Stephanie Kellington (2001). 'Changing the Balance of Power: The Listen Up! Research Project and Participatory Research in Marginalized Communities'. Paper prepared for the Commonwealth Secretariat/Maritime Centre of Excellence for Women's Health co-publication.

UNAIDS (1997). *Women and AIDS: UNAIDS Point of View*. Geneva: Joint United Nations Programme on HIV/AIDS.

—— (1999). *Gender and HIV/AIDS: Taking Stock of Research and Programmes*. Geneva: Joint United Nations Programme on HIV/AIDS.

—— (2001a). *Resource Packet on Gender & AIDS*. Los Altos: Sociometrics.

—— (2001b). *Together We Can: Leadership in a World of AIDS*. Geneva: Joint United Nations Programme on HIV/AIDS.

UNAIDS/WHO (2001). *AIDS Epidemic Update: December 2001*. Geneva: UNAIDS and WHO.

UNDPI and UNAIDS (2001). *Fact Sheets: Global Crisis … Global Action*. New York: UNDPI and UNAIDS.

UNFPA (2000a). 'Gender and HIV/AIDS: Leadership Roles in Social Mobilization'. Report of the UNFPA-organised break-out panel, African Development Forum, Addis Ababa, 3–7 December.

—— (2000b). *The State of the World Population – Lives Together, Worlds Apart: Men and women in a time of change*. New York: United Nations Population Fund.

—— (nd). *Preventing Infection; Promoting Reproductive Health:*

UNFPA's Response to HIV/AIDS. New York: UNFPA.

UNICEF (2000). *The Progress of Nations 2000.* New York: UNICEF.

UNICEF (2001). Young People and HIV/AIDS. A UNICEF Fact Sheet. New York: UNICEF.

UNIFEM, WHO and UNAIDS (2000). 'The HIV/AIDS pandemic and its gender implications'. Report of the UN Expert Group Meeting on Gender and HIV/AIDS, Windhoek, Namibia, 13–17 November.

UNIFEM (2001). 'Women, Gender and HIV/AIDS in East and Southeast Asia'. Information pack distributed at the 45th Session of the UN Commission on the Status of Women, New York, 6–16 March.

United Nations (1999). 'Thematic Issues Before the Commission on the Status of Women: Report of the Secretary-General'. E/CN.6/1999/4. New York: United Nations.

—— (2000). 'Security Council Resolution on Women, Peace and Security'. S/2000/1044. New York: United Nations.

Welbourn, Alice (1999). 'Gender, Sex and HIV: How to address issues that no-one wants to hear about'. In Yvonne Preiswerk (ed.). *Tant qu'on a la santé: les determinants socio-économiques et culturels de la santé dans les relations sociales entre les femmes et les hommes.* Berne: UNESCO.

WHO (2000a). *Violence against Women.* Fact Sheet No. 239. Geneva: World Health Organization.

—— (2000b). *Human Rights, Women and HIV/AIDS.* Fact Sheet No. 247. Geneva: World Health Organization.

—— /UNICEF (1994). *Action for Children Affected with AIDS: Programme profiles and lessons learned.* New York: UNICEF.

Whynot, Elizabeth (1998). 'Women who use injection drugs: The social context of risk'. In *Canadian Medical Association Journal,* 159: 355–8.

Women & Environments International (2000) Issue 48/49, Summer/Fall. (http://www.utoronto.ca/iwsgs/we.mag)

Appendix 1: UN Guidelines on HIV-related Human Rights

Guideline 1
States should establish an effective national framework for their response to HIV/AIDS which ensures a co-ordinated, participatory, transparent and accountable approach, integrating HIV/AIDS policy and programme responsibilities across all branches of government.

Guideline 2
States should ensure, through political and financial support, that community consultation occurs in all phases of HIV/AIDS policy design, programme implementation and evaluation and that community organisations are enabled to carry out their activities, including in the field of ethics, law and human rights, effectively.

Guideline 3
States should review and reform public health laws to ensure that they adequately address public health issues raised by HIV/AIDS, that their provisions applicable to casually transmitted diseases are not inappropriately applied to HIV/AIDS and that they are consistent with international human rights obligations.

Guideline 4
States should review and reform criminal laws and correctional systems to ensure that they are consistent with international human rights obligations and are not misused in the context of HIV/AIDS or targeted against vulnerable groups.

Guideline 5
States should enact or strengthen anti-discrimination and other protective laws that protect vulnerable groups, people living with HIV/AIDS and people with disabilities from discrimination in both the public and private sectors, ensure pri-

vacy and confidentiality and ethics in research involving human subjects, emphasise education and conciliation,

Guideline 6

States should enact legislation to provide for the regulation of HIV-related goods, services and information, so as to ensure widespread availability of qualitative prevention measures and services, adequate HIV prevention and care information and safe and effective medication at an affordable price.

Guideline 7

States should implement and support legal support services that will educate people affected by HIV/AIDS about their rights, provide free legal services to enforce those rights, develop expertise on HIV-related legal issues and utilise means of protection in addition to the courts, such as offices of ministries of justice, ombudspersons, health complaint units and human rights commissions.

Guideline 8

States, in collaboration with and through the community, should promote a supportive and enabling environment for women, children and other vulnerable groups by addressing underlying prejudices and inequalities through community dialogue, specially designed social and health services and support to community groups.

Guideline 9

States should promote the wide and ongoing distribution of creative education, training and media programmes explicitly designed to change attitudes of discrimination and stigmatisation associated with HIV/AIDS to understanding and acceptance.

Guideline 10

States should ensure that government and the private sector develop codes of conduct regarding HIV/AIDS issues that translate human rights principles into codes of professional responsibility and practice, with accompanying mechanisms to implement and enforce these codes.

Guideline 11

States should ensure monitoring and enforcement mechanisms to guarantee the protection of HIV-related human rights, including those of people living with HIV/AIDS, their families and communities.

Guideline 12

States should co-operate through all relevant programmes and agencies of the United Nations system, including UNAIDS, to share knowledge and experience concerning HIV-related human rights issues and should ensure effective mechanisms to protect human rights in the context of HIV/AIDS at international level.

Source: OHCHR and UNAIDS, 1996

Appendix 2: Global and Commonwealth Mandates on Gender and HIV/AIDS

Global Mandates

The Convention for the Elimination of all forms of Discrimination Against Women (CEDAW) (1981)

This convention has been ratified by 166 states at the time of writing, including most members of the Commonwealth. In article 1, it defines discrimination against women as: 'any distinction, exclusion or restriction made on the basis of sex which has the effect or purpose of impairing or nullifying the recognition, enjoyment or exercise by women, irrespective of their marital status, on a basis of equality of men and women, of human rights and fundamental freedoms in the political, economic, social, cultural, civil or any other field'. This definition has been accepted by the Human Rights Committee as applicable to discrimination under the International Covenant on Civil and Political Rights (ICCPR).

Article 12 of the convention is concerned with the area of health. HIV/AIDS is not specifically addressed since there was not a global pandemic at the time the convention came into force. However, it is the focus of General Recommendation 15: 'Avoidance of Discrimination against Women in National Strategies for the Prevention and Control of AIDS' (1990).[3] This recommends that State Parties:

- make information more widely available to increase public awareness of the risk and effects of HIV infection and AIDS, especially to women and children;

---

[3] The Committee on the Elimination of Discrimination Against Women (CEDAW) has made a number of General Recommendations. Although these are not a formally binding interpretation of the Convention, they 'have considerable authority … [and should] be an integral part of the domestic application of international law' (Bayefsky, 1994).

- ensure that AIDS programmes give special attention to the rights and needs of women and children, and to the ways in which the reproductive role of women and their subordinate position in some societies makes them especially vulnerable to HIV infection;

- take measures to ensure the active participation of women in primary health care and to enhance their role as care providers, health workers and educators in the prevention of infection with HIV;

- include information in their reports under article 12 of the Convention on the effects of AIDS on the situation of women and on the action taken to cater to the needs of those women who are infected and to prevent specific discrimination against them.

At its 14th (1996), 16th (1997), 18th (1998), 20th (1999) and 22nd and 23rd (2000) sessions, the Committee expressed its concern about the effect of the HIV/AIDS pandemic on young women in a number of contexts. These include prostitution, trafficking in women and girls, health education, lack of statistical data on HIV/AIDS – including sex-disaggregated data – and risks of parent-to-child transmission. The Committee therefore recommended:

- more information on the prevention of HIV/AIDS;

- more studies and statistical data;

- access of prostitutes to appropriate health service;

- education in sexual and reproductive health, including HIV/AIDS;

- promotion of condom use; and

- increased education and services on HIV/AIDS to all women, including rural women.

Programme of Action of the International Conference on Population and Development (ICPD, Cairo, 1994)

At the 1994 International Conference on Population and Development (ICPD), held in Cairo, 179 countries agreed that population and development are inextricably linked, and that empowering women and meeting people's needs for education and health, including reproductive health, are necessary for both individual advancement and balanced development. The Programme of Action (PoA) identifies advancing gender equality and equity and the empowerment of women, the elimination of all kinds of violence against women and ensuring women's ability to control their own fertility as cornerstones of population and development-related programmes (principle 4).

Sexually transmitted infections (STIs)

Section C recommends actions designed to prevent, reduce the incidence of and provide treatment for STIs, including HIV/AIDS. Such actions include to:

- increase efforts in reproductive health programmes to prevent, detect and treat STIs and other reproductive tract infections;

- provide specialised training to all health-care providers in the prevention and detection of, and counselling on, STIs, especially infections in women and youth;

- make information, counselling for responsible sexual behaviour and effective prevention of STIs and HIV integral components of all reproductive and sexual health services; and

- promote and distribute high-quality condoms as integral components of all reproductive health-care services (para. 7.30–33).

The AIDS pandemic

Section D calls on governments to mobilise all segments of society to control the AIDS pandemic. Actions include to:

- provide sex education and information to both those infected and those not infected, and especially to adolescents;

- ensure health providers have training in:

  - promoting responsible sexual behaviour, including voluntary sexual abstinence and condom use, in education and information programmes;

Box 23: Benchmark Indicators Adopted at the ICPD +5 Review

After reviewing progress made in the goals and objectives set by the ICPD Programme of Action (1994), the 1999 General Assembly special session (ICPD +5) agreed on a new set of benchmarks. These included:

- By 2005, 60 per cent of primary health care and family planning facilities should offer the widest achievable range of safe and effective family planning methods, essential obstetric care, prevention and management of reproductive tract infections, including sexually transmitted diseases, and barrier methods to prevent infection. By 2010, 80 per cent of facilities should offer such services and by 2015 all should do so.

- By 2005, the gap between the proportion of individuals using contraceptives and the proportion expressing a desire to space or limit their families should be reduced by half, by 2010 by 75 per cent, and by 2015 by 100 per cent. Recruitment targets or quotas should not be used in attempting to reach this goal.

- By 2005, at least 90 per cent of young men and women aged 15–24 should have access to preventive methods to reduce vulnerability to HIV/AIDS infection – such as female and male condoms, voluntary testing, counselling and follow up, and by 2010 at least 95 per cent.

- By 2005, HIV infection rates in young people aged 15–24 should be reduced by 25 per cent in the most affected countries and by 2010 by 25 per cent globally.

Source: www.unfpa.org/icpd/index.htm

- counselling on sexually transmitted diseases and HIV infection, including the assessment and identification of high-risk behaviours needing special attention and services;

- the avoidance of contaminated equipment and blood products; and

- the avoidance of sharing needles among injecting drug users;

- develop guidelines and counselling services on AIDS and STIs within the primary health-care services;

- mobilise all segments of society to control the AIDS pandemic, including NGOs, community organisations, religious leaders, the private sector, the media, schools and health facilities;

- develop policies and guidelines to protect the individual rights of and eliminate discrimination against persons infected with HIV and their families;

- devise special programmes to provide care and the necessary emotional support to men and women affected by AIDS and to counsel their families and near relations;

- promote responsible sexual behaviour, including voluntary sexual abstinence, for the prevention of HIV infection;

- make condoms and drugs for the prevention and treatment of STIs widely available and affordable and included in all essential drug lists; and

- further control the quality of blood products and equipment decontamination (paras. 8.30–35).

A 1999 review of progress since the Cairo Conference culminated in a Special Session of the United Nations General Assembly (ICPD +5) which identified key actions needed for further implementation of the PoA and new benchmarks for measuring progress towards ICPD goals (see Box 23).

Beijing Declaration and Platform for Action, Fourth World Conference on Women (1995)

Participants: All Commonwealth countries, either in national delegations or through the Commonwealth Secretariat.

The Beijing Platform for Action (PFA) identifies five strategic objectives in the area of health, under each of which governments agreed to take a number of actions. Objective C3 calls for gender-sensitive initiatives that address STIs, HIV/

AIDS, and sexual and reproductive health issues. Actions to be taken include to:

- ensure the involvement of women, especially those infected with HIV/AIDS or other STIs or affected by the HIV/AIDS pandemic, in all decision-making relating to the development, implementation, monitoring and evaluation of policies and programmes on HIV/AIDS and other STIs;

- review and amend laws and combat practices that may contribute to women's susceptibility to HIV infection and other STIs;

- encourage all sectors of society to develop compassionate and supportive, non-discriminatory HIV/AIDS-related policies and practices that protect the rights of infected individuals;

- develop gender-sensitive multisectoral programmes and strategies to end the social subordination of women and girls and to ensure their social and economic empowerment and equality;

- support and strengthen national capacity to create and improve gender-sensitive policies and programmes on HIV/AIDS and other STIs;

- provide workshops and specialised education and training to parents, decision makers and opinion leaders at all levels of the community, including religious and traditional authorities, on prevention of HIV/AIDS and other STIs and on their effect on both women and men of all ages;

- give full attention to the promotion of mutually respectful and equitable gender relations and, in particular, to meeting the educational and service needs of adolescents to enable them to deal in a positive and responsible way with their sexuality;

- design specific programmes for men of all ages and male adolescents aimed at providing complete and accurate information on safe and responsible sexual and reproductive behaviour, and educate and enable men to assume their responsibilities to prevent HIV/AIDS and other STIs;

- ensure the provision, through the primary health-care system, of universal access of couples and individuals to appropriate and affordable preventive services with respect to STIs, including HIV/AIDS; and

- support and expedite action-oriented research on affordable methods, controlled by women, to prevent HIV and other STIs, and on methods of care, support and treatment of women, ensuring their involvement in all aspects of such research (para. 108).

Beijing +5 Outcome Document (2000)

Five years after Beijing, governments met in New York at a Special Session of the General Assembly entitled 'Women 2000: Gender Equality, Development and Peace for the Twenty-first Century' (popularly known as Beijing +5). Governments adopted the 'Further Actions and Initiatives to Implement the Beijing Declaration and the Platform for Action (PFA)' by which they reaffirmed their commitment to the goals and objectives contained in the Beijing Declaration and PFA and to the implementation of the 12 critical areas of concern. In the area of HIV/AIDS, they also agreed to undertake a number of further actions, including to:

- Adopt policies and implement measures to address the gender aspects of health challenges such as HIV/AIDS (para. 72a).

- Give priority attention to measures to prevent, detect and treat STIs, including HIV/AIDS (para. 72b).

- Revise national policies, programmes and legislation to implement the key actions for the further implementation of the ICPD Programme of Action. Particular attention should be paid to providing a wide range of safe and effective family planning and contraceptive methods; and reducing young people's risk of HIV/AIDS (para. 79c).

- Promote people's right to make decisions concerning reproduction free of discrimination, coercion and violence (para. 72j).

- Promote mutually respectful and equitable gender relations (para. 72j).

- Design and implement programmes for adolescents with their full involvement to provide them with education, information and appropriate, specific, user-friendly and accessible services that address their reproductive and sexual health needs (para. 79f).

- Design and implement programmes to encourage and enable men to adopt safe and responsible sexual and reproductive behaviour, and to effectively use methods to prevent unwanted pregnancies and STIs, including HIV/AIDS (para. 72l).

- Adopt measures to ensure non-discrimination against and respect for the privacy of those living with HIV/AIDS and STIs, including women and young people. They should have access to the information needed to prevent further transmission of HIV/AIDS and STIs and be able to access treatment and care services without fear of stigmatisation, discrimination or violence (para. 72n).

- Encourage a high awareness of the harmful effects of certain traditional or customary practices affecting the health of women, some of which increase their vulnerability to HIV/AIDS and other STIs, and intensify efforts to eliminate such practices (para. 98d).

- Intensify education, services and community-based mobilisation strategies to protect women of all ages from HIV and other STIs. This should include:

  - the development of safe, affordable, effective and easily accessible female-controlled methods, including microbicides and female condoms;

  - voluntary and confidential HIV testing and counselling;

  - the promotion of responsible sexual behaviour, including abstinence and condom use;

  - the development of vaccines, simple low-cost diagnosis and single dose treatments for sexually transmitted infections (para. 103b).

- Provide access to adequate and affordable treatment, monitoring and care for all people, especially women and girls, infected with STIs or living with life-threatening diseases, including HIV/AIDS and associated opportunistic infections, such as tuberculosis (para. 103c).

- Provide gender-sensitive support systems for women and other family members who are involved in caring for persons affected by serious health conditions, including HIV/AIDS (para. 103c).

- Eliminate gender biases in bio-medical, clinical and social research. This includes conducting voluntary clinical trials involving women, with due regard for their human rights, and gathering, analysing and making available to appropriate institutions and to end-users gender-specific information about dosage, side-effects and effectiveness of drugs, including contraceptives and methods that protect against STIs (para. 92d).

- Promote, improve, systemise and fund the collection of data disaggregated by sex, age and other appropriate factors, on health and access to health services, including comprehensive information on the impact of HIV/AIDS on women, throughout the life-cycle (para. 92c).

Declaration of Commitment on HIV/AIDS, 'Global Crisis – Global Action', Special Session of the UN General Assembly on the Problem of HIV/AIDS in All its Aspects (2001)

A Special Session of the UN General Assembly was held in June 2001 in order to intensify international action to fight the HIV/AIDS epidemic and to mobilise the resources needed. Governments unanimously agreed on a Declaration of Commitment to reduce infection rates by 25 per cent by 2005, end discrimination by challenging 'gender stereotypes and attitudes' and inequalities between men and women worldwide, and provide AIDS education to 90 per cent of young people by 2005. Poverty, women's rights and funding issues were also addressed as a part of the solution to combat HIV/AIDS.

In the Declaration, governments emphasise that the vulnerable must be given priority in the response to the HIV/AIDS crisis, and that empowering women is essential for reducing vulnerability. They agree to take action in eleven key areas:

- Leadership

- Prevention

- Care, support and treatment

- HIV/AIDS and human rights

- Reducing vulnerability

- Children orphaned and made vulnerable by HIV/AIDS

- Alleviating social and economic impact

- Research and development

- HIV/AIDS in conflict and disaster affected regions

- Resources

- Follow up.

All countries are called on to take the necessary steps to implement, in "strengthened partnership and co-operation with other multilateral and bilateral partners and with civil society", a number of time-bound targets, including to:

By 2003
- Ensure the development and implementation of multisectoral national strategies and financing plans for combating HIV/AIDS that:

  - address the epidemic in forthright terms;

  - confront stigma, silence and denial;

  - address gender and age-based dimensions of the epidemic;

  - eliminate discrimination and marginalisation;

  - involve partnerships with civil society and the business sector and the full participation of people living with HIV/AIDS, those in vulnerable groups and people mostly at risk, particularly women and young people;

- are resourced to the extent possible from national budgets;

- fully promote and protect all human rights and fundamental freedoms, including the right to the highest attainable standard of physical and mental health;

- integrate a gender perspective;

- address risk, vulnerability, prevention, care, treatment and support and reduction of the impact of the epidemic; and strengthen health, education and legal system capacity (para. 37).

- Establish time-bound national targets to achieve the internationally agreed goal of reducing HIV prevalence among young men and women aged 15–24 by 25 per cent in the most affected countries by 2005 and globally by 2010. Intensify efforts to achieve these targets as well as to challenge gender stereotypes and attitudes and gender inequalities in relation to HIV/AIDS, encouraging the active involvement of men and boys (para. 47).

- Have in place in all countries strategies, policies and programmes that identify and begin to address those factors that make individuals particularly vulnerable to HIV infection, including:

  - underdevelopment

  - economic insecurity

  - poverty

  - lack of empowerment of women

  - lack of education

  - social exclusion

  - illiteracy

  - discrimination

  - lack of information and/or commodities for self-protection

  - all types of sexual exploitation of women, girls and boys, including for commercial reasons.

Such strategies, policies and programmes should address the gender dimension of the epidemic, specify the action that will be taken to address vulnerability and set targets for achievement (para. 62).

- Develop and/or strengthen strategies, policies and programmes to reduce the vulnerability of children and young people by ensuring their access to primary and secondary education; including HIV/AIDS in curricula for adolescents; and ensuring safe and secure environments, especially for young girls (para. 63).

- Evaluate the economic and social impact of the HIV/AIDS epidemic and develop multisectoral strategies to:

  - address the impact at the individual, family, community and national levels;

  - develop and accelerate the implementation of national poverty eradication strategies to address the impact of HIV/AIDS on household income, livelihoods, and access to basic social services, with a special focus on individuals, families and communities severely affected by the epidemic; and

  - review the social and economic impact of HIV/AIDS at all levels of society especially on women and the elderly, particularly in their role as caregivers and in families affected by HIV/AIDS and address their special needs (para. 68).

- Develop and begin to implement national strategies that incorporate HIV/AIDS awareness, prevention, care and treatment elements into programmes or actions that respond to emergency situations. Populations destabilised by armed conflict, humanitarian emergencies and natural disasters, particularly women and children, are at increased risk of exposure to HIV infection (para. 75).

By 2005
- Ensure that a wide range of prevention programmes is available in all countries, including:

  - information, education and communication aimed at

reducing risk-taking behaviour and encouraging responsible sexual behaviour, including abstinence and fidelity;

- expanded access to essential commodities, including male and female condoms; and

- early and effective treatment of sexually transmittable infections (para. 52).

- Ensure that at least 90 per cent, and by 2010 at least 95 per cent, of young men and women aged 15–24 have access to the information and education necessary to develop the life skills required to reduce their vulnerability to HIV infection (para. 53).

- Reduce the proportion of infants infected with HIV by 20 per cent, and by 50 per cent by 2010, by:

  - ensuring that 80 per cent of pregnant women accessing antenatal care have information, counselling and other HIV prevention services available to them;

  - increasing the availability of effective treatment to reduce mother-to-child transmission of HIV;

  - providing effective interventions for HIV-infected women (para. 54).

- Implement national strategies that:

  - promote the advancement of women and women's full enjoyment of all human rights;

  - promote shared responsibility of men and women to ensure safe sex;

  - empower women to have control over and decide freely and responsibly on matters related to their sexuality to increase their ability to protect themselves from HIV infection (para. 59).

- Implement measures to increase capacities of women and adolescent girls to protect themselves from the risk of HIV infection through:

  - the provision of health care and health services, including sexual and reproductive health;

- prevention education that promotes gender equality within a culturally and gender sensitive framework (para. 60).

- Ensure development and accelerated implementation of national strategies for women's empowerment; promotion and protection of women's full enjoyment of all human rights; and reduction of their vulnerability to HIV/AIDS. This should include the elimination of all forms of discrimination, as well as all forms of violence against women and girls, including harmful traditional and customary practices, abuse, rape and other forms of sexual violence, battering and trafficking in women and girls (para. 61).

Periodically
Conduct national reviews involving the participation of civil society, particularly people living with HIV/AIDS, vulnerable groups and caregivers, of progress achieved in realising these commitments and identify problems and obstacles to achieving progress and ensure wide dissemination of the results of these reviews (para. 94).

Commonwealth Mandates

Commonwealth Plan of Action on Gender and Development (1995) and its Update (2000–2005)

Signatories: All Commonwealth Heads of Government

The 1995 Commonwealth Plan of Action on Gender and Development and its Update are a blueprint for Commonwealth action to achieve gender equality. The Plan states as its vision that the Commonwealth works towards a world in which women and men have equal rights and opportunities at all stages of their lives to express their creativity in all fields of human endeavour. This world is also one in which women are respected and valued as equal and able partners in establishing values of social justice, equity, democracy and respect for human rights. Within such a framework of values, women and men will work in collaboration and partnership to ensure people-centred sustainable development for all nations (4.1.1).

To achieve this vision, the Commonwealth member governments will put in place national action plans with a key focus on strengthening institutional capacity. Fifteen elements are identified as desirable components for national action plans, including:

- Integrate gender issues in all national policies, plans and programmes.

- Promote equal opportunities and positive and/or affirmative action throughout the country and consult women on priorities.

- Action for anti-discrimination.

- Women's rights as human rights, the elimination of violence against women, the protection of the girls child and the outlawing of all forms of trafficking in women and girls.

- Action for women's participation in decision-making.

- Action for sustainable development, poverty alleviation and eradication of absolute poverty.

- Action for human resource development, literacy, training and education.

- Action for women's health. This includes increasing women's access to affordable, quality health care and related services that meet their needs and priorities, and ensure their full participation as decision-makers in the development and design of health policies and programmes that impact on their lives and those of their families and communities. Empower women to protect and care for themselves, particularly in relation to maternal and infant mortality, HIV/AIDS and other infectious diseases.

Commonwealth Heads of Government Meeting (CHOGM) Mandates (1999)

Heads of government at the 1999 CHOGM expressed grave concern over the devastating social and economic impact of HIV/AIDS, particularly in sub-Saharan Africa. They agreed that this constituted a Global Emergency and pledged personally to lead the fight against HIV/AIDS within their countries and internationally. They urged all sectors in government, international agencies and the private sector to co-operate in increased efforts to tackle the problem (para. 55, 1999 Durban CHOGM Communiqué).